The nMRCGP H[a...]
2nd edition

By

Dr Bob Mortimer

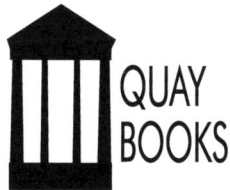

QUAY
BOOKS

A division of MA Healthcare Ltd

Quay Books Division, MA Healthcare Ltd, St Jude's Church, Dulwich Road, London SE24 0PB

British Library Cataloguing-in-Publication Data
A catalogue record is available for this book

© MA Healthcare Limited 2009
1st edition September 2007
ISBN-10: 1-85642-383-2
ISBN-13: 978-1-85642-383-0

Printed in the UK by CLE, St Ives, Huntingdon, Cambridgeshire

Contents

About the author

Dr Bob Mortimer qualified from the Welsh National School of Medicine, Cardiff, in 1983. He passed the MRCGP in 1992, and became a Fellow of the Royal College of General Practitioners in 2005. He has been a GP trainer since 1995. In 1994 he set up the Swansea MRCGP Course and became an examiner in 1996, obtaining the Diploma in Medical Education (Cardiff) in 1998. Dr Mortimer was Associate Director for the Welsh Deanery until 2005.

Dr Mortimer is a full time GP and is an assessor for the Clinical Skills Assessment (CSA), and in addition to being a trainer for assessors he is also one of the senior marshals involved in the actual running of the CSA. He also runs the Swansea MRCGP Course.

Acknowledgements

I would like to thank the Panel of Examiners for the MRCGP Examination, who have been the most inspiring group of people I have ever had the privilege to work with.

Foreword to the second edition

I am retired now and I still dream of failing finals. I also dream of the little man knocking at my door and saying: *'Found you out, you are a fake aren't you'*. That is the trouble with exams, they are both memorable and important. I still remember my viva for the MRCGP in 1974 because it was searching, relevant and it found me out — not quite enough to fail, but enough to tell me that my learning was nowhere near done.

The MRCGP exam became part of my own life, and after 25 years as an examiner I retired as Convenor just as the old exam metamorphosed into the new. The nMRCGP exam, unlike the old MRCGP, is a licensing exam. This means that it is not an optional extra but an essential requirement to be a primary care doctor. It marks the end of your initial training.

General practice remains one of the hardest of all medical disciplines to do well: it requires a complex synthesis of knowledge, curiosity, tenacity and humanity. Over the last 60 years general practitioners have often been derided by more specialised colleagues as academically slightly below par; in some cases this was true, but for most patients it is the skill of the generalist that is needed by the specialist as much as the other way round. These arguments have become less heated and less relevant, but such attitudes are still around in hospitals and medical schools.

This book is about the academic underpinning of the discipline you have chosen. You owe it to your patients and to yourself to practise general medicine to the best of your knowledge and ability. This of course means not just passing the nMRCGP, but also learning how to learn and keep learning. This book will enable you to catch a glimpse of the thinking of the generations of general practitioners who have contributed to the development of the examination.

Bob Mortimer has produced a straightforward, easy-to-read book that gives you all the information to help you surmount this hurdle in your life without too much difficulty. The exam is modern, very wide ranging, searching and stimulating — yes, stimulating! This wonderful little book tells you all you need to know about the examination, its ethos and its methods. It is written by a good friend who is an examiner of many years standing and a working GP. I am able to hear Bob's voice as I read the text. You will find it full of good advice, spot-on up-to-date information, technical tips, and inside knowledge, but to me the best of all is the humanity, wisdom and experience of the author that illuminates the whole. This is not just a book about how to pass an exam, but is a manual to help you learn for a whole career.

Dr Peter Tate MBE FRCGP
Retired Convenor MRCGP Examination

Foreword to the first edition

I never enjoyed taking exams. Who does? But several decades ago, when I was coming to the end of my vocational training as a fledgling GP, I took the Membership of the Royal College of General Practitioners (MRCGP) Examination. I have never been a good judge of how I was doing during exams, and my pessimism was often justified. On this occasion I thought I was floundering. None of the questions had seemed straightforward, and my doubts and insecurity were increasing by the minute. And so, when the examiner asked me how I would deal with a patient who had been bitten by a dog shortly before boarding a plane in India the previous day, I just shrugged. '*I'm sorry*', I said despairingly, '*I just don't know anything at all about rabies. I'd look it up*'.

But instead of groaning, both examiners grinned. One said: '*I've been asking this question for five days. You're the first one to give me the right answer*'.

And he was not joking. For a UK family doctor to treat possible rabies from memory would indeed be unsafe and unwise. Ultimately my result was better than I had ever dreamt of, and I decided this was a 'real-world' organisation that I could do business with. All too many examinations in the past seemed to have been built on theory alone. The Royal College of General Practitioners (RCGP) seemed to me to focus on the uncertain and unpredictable world that real GPs face with real patients, and over many years working with the RCGP, including 15 years as an examiner, my view has not changed.

That was then. This is now. The arrival of the Postgraduate Medical Education Training Board has led to the introduction of new curricula across every medical specialty, providing common standards, clarity and transparency to training, as well as promoting the continuous development of doctors' skills in order to meet patient need. General Practice, at long last, has now been recognised as a medical specialty equivalent to every other, and new assessment methodologies have been developed to match.

But change is always rather confusing, and it certainly feels threatening for learners as well as their trainers. At this time of great change in the MRCGP Examination, this book offers real insight and real support. Quite rightly, it stresses that the best way of passing the exam is by becoming a good GP. Exam technique, and understanding how exams work is important, but nothing counts for as much as being a caring, learning, and listening GP.

The nMRCGP is now a licensing exam. Every new GP in the UK will have to pass it. This is exactly how it should be — after all, being a GP is one of the most complex and skilled jobs in medicine, and it has always seemed insulting that lower mandatory standards were acceptable in our specialty. But now they are not. You have to pass, and the nation's patients deserve nothing less.

Reading this beautifully written, informative and supportive book will demystify many of the changes in the nMRCGP exam, and allows the reader to focus on what really matters — the patients and the care we can offer. High quality General Practice is of vital importance to patients everywhere. After all, good GPs really do make a difference.

Professor David Haslam CBE, FRCP, FFPH, PRCGP
President of the Royal College of General Practitioners

CHAPTER I

Why do we need exams?

The aim of this book is to help you prepare for and pass the new membership exam for the Royal College of General Practitioners — the *n*MRCGP. This introduction will explain why the exam is there and how it came about. It might not seem terribly relevant to you right now, but the key to passing any examination is to get to know as much about it as you can.

This book will describe the elements of the exam in some detail, with information on what each part is designed to assess and the methods used to assess you. There will be lots of practical advice on how you should prepare for the exam and how to ensure your best performance on the day.

There are no easy shortcuts to passing the *n*MRCGP, it is a highly rigorous assessment of your knowledge, clinical and communication skills and your ability to solve problems in general practice. Making sure you understand the exam will however mean that you can make efficient use of your time preparing for it. Much of your learning for the exam can be within your day-to-day experiences in your work, and this book will, wherever possible, advise you on how to maximise the benefit you gain from these experiences and minimise the amount of the more traditional, and often less interesting, methods of preparing for an exam such as reading textbooks and journals. You will of course need to do some reading for the exam, but this book will help you to target the right material and use it efficiently.

Reasons for exams generally

By the time you get to sit the *n*MRCGP you will be quite an exam expert. You will have taken GCSEs at age 16 (or their equivalent where you were educated), A-levels or equivalent at age 18, followed by the various hurdles set in your way throughout medical school. Generally speaking the degree of difficulty rises as you progress through your career. There are several reasons for exams existing:

- To ensure suitability or ability to pursue a particular course of study — for example the assessment used for entry into training for general practice
- To check that you have learned what you were supposed to in your coursework

- To discriminate between applicants for a job or a place in a school or college
- To ensure you have the knowledge and skills required to do a particular job
- As a mark of status, or to demonstrate a level of excellence.

When you sit an exam it is important to have a clear idea of why you are taking it and what it is there to test. The previous MRCGP examination was mainly aimed at the last of the above bullet points — a pass demonstrated that you had achieved a level of excellence. It was also to some extent used to discriminate, for example practices appointing a new partner or salaried doctor would usually prefer someone who had passed the MRCGP exam and it was generally required if you wanted to become a GP trainer.

The new assessment however is a *licensing* examination and its main purpose is to ensure that you are fit to practice as an independent, unsupervised GP in the UK.

Over the last few decades general practice in the UK has undergone dramatic change. It is just as demanding a career as any other in medicine and is no longer, if indeed it ever was, a 'soft option' compared to the medical and surgical specialties. A GP requires a working knowledge of all areas of medicine, surgery, paediatrics, gynaecology, etc. and needs advanced communication and clinical skills to apply this knowledge. GPs must be able to work in complex multi-disciplinary teams, often in a lead role, and have significant responsibilities in managing access to secondary care. Once you are qualified as a GP you have to do all this independently and without supervision, although most of us are fortunate enough to work in supportive practice environments.

Another issue is the effect a rigorous entrance examination has on the perception of a profession by others — setting a meaningful minimum standard for general practice can only enhance its standing both with the general public and with our peers in other specialties. This then has a knock-on effect on morale within the profession leading to enhanced self-esteem among GPs along with improved recruitment.

Exams can test various things:

- Recall of facts you are supposed to have learned
- Ability to reason and solve problems
- Practical skills
- Checking some of your values and attitudes.

There are many different types of exams, and each type of exam will be more or less effective at assessing each of these attributes. The modules of the *n*MRCGP are designed to ensure that they rigorously assess all of the above and we will explore which module assesses which attributes throughout this book.

The history of the MRCGP examination

The MRCGP has always been the examination to gain *membership* of the Royal College of General Practitioners (RCGP). Until 1968 a GP could join the College by simply paying a fee. Then along came the Membership exam and this became the only route to College membership. You did not *need* to become a member of the RCGP, and historically only just over half of trainee GPs took the exam and became members.

Those who did take the exam did so for various reasons — some because they felt it was important to be a member of the College, but these were probably in the minority. Some took the exam as a personal challenge and as an affirmation that they had attained a certain level of achievement following their vocational training. Some did it out of peer pressure or because their course organiser or trainer expected them to do it. Probably the largest group was those who did it because they thought it might improve their chances in job applications.

Initially the MRCGP comprised a multiple choice question paper (MCQ), a modified essay question paper (MEQ), a practice topic question paper (PTQ) and two oral examinations. Over the years these were gradually refined, often as a result of analysis and advice from the College's psychometric advisers. For example, over time the MCQ stopped using negative marking as this discriminated against more timid candidates who were afraid to guess, and the true/false question format developed into extended matching questions and other question formats as this increased its ability to accurately discriminate between strong and weak candidates. Many of the lessons learned from this development have been incorporated into the new assessment and the College continues to work with psychometric experts to ensure its robustness.

About the *n*MRCGP examination

Until 2007, GP registrars in the UK had to satisfy the requirements of the Joint Committee on Postgraduate Training for General Practice (JCPTGP) by passing Summative Assessment. Some of the elements of Summative Assessment could be exempted by passing the appropriate modules of the MRCGP examination. At this time the Government replaced the JCPTGP with a new body called the Postgraduate Medical Education and Training Board (PMETB, generally pronounced *pee-met-bee*). While the JCPTGP oversaw only training for general practice, the PMETB has responsibility for all the medical specialties. The JCPTGP was called the Joint Committee as it was made up of representatives from both the Royal College of GPs and the General Practitioners Committee of the British Medical Association (BMA) (i.e. from the profession's academic body as well as from its 'trade union'). The vast majority of its members were GPs.

The PMETB is entirely different, with its members appointed by government and with 17 medical members (four of whom have a background in general practice) and eight lay members. It was decided that there was to be a new licensing examination for each medical specialty, and that this would be approved and overseen by the PMETB (Department of Health [DH], 2001).

The RCGP followed these political developments closely and from an early stage started planning the new assessment. It was clear that any new assessment would need to be specifically designed to assess GP registrars at the end of training, and that simply presenting the existing exam would not be acceptable. The College has developed its curriculum for general practice and this formed the basis for the new assessment which was designed to ensure that it tested all areas within the curriculum. For each area of the curriculum it was considered what form of test would be most fit for purpose. The RCGP curriculum will be covered in the next chapter.

The key challenges to the new examination were developing an assessment that was rigorous and robust enough to stand up to legal challenge; that had more emphasis than previous assessments on doctors' practical skills in consulting with and examining patients, and that assessed their progress through their training in a more structured and rigorous way. It also had to be able to assess the 3,000 or so doctors completing GP training each year.

There was a lot of discussion about the actual standard that was to be set — the MRCGP had previously had an overall pass rate of just over 70% while only a handful of doctors failed Summative Assessment each year. On the one hand it was felt that a pass rate of 98–99% was inappropriately high and would be allowing through doctors who almost certainly had not achieved a high enough level of competence, and it was also accepted that the implications of preventing almost 30% of registrars from entering general practice immediately after training were significant. Therefore it was important from the outset that the new assessment must be *criterion referenced*, meaning that it made an objective assessment of a doctor without comparison to everyone else taking the assessment. This makes standard setting even more important since it means that theoretically the assessment could fail everyone who took it if the standard were set too high, or conversely pass everyone if it were too low.

The development of the new assessment has been led by various working groups comprised of members from both the College and the Deaneries across the UK, as well as having extensive input from lay representatives. The final product has three components:

- An applied knowledge test (AKT), which is a multiple choice type test
- The clinical skills assessment (CSA), which is a series of consultations with simulated patients.
- The workplace based assessment (WPBA), which is a structured assessment of the registrar's work in their training practice.

The responsibility for the AKT and the CSA is largely held by the RCGP, with the Deaneries largely responsible for the WPBA, The *e*Portfolio is run by the College.

A registrar will not 'qualify' as a GP until they have satisfactorily completed all three components (AKT, CSA, and WPBA). The workplace based assessment is continuous throughout the three years of training (see Chapter 4). The applied knowledge test can be taken at any time during training but will usually take place during the last year of training, and the clinical skills assessment will need to be taken during the last year in general practice training.

The applied knowledge test

From the outset the applied knowledge test has been closely based on the 'old' MRCGP multiple choice question paper and the new test was developed by the same group of examiners. There is little dispute that the multiple choice question format is best suited to reliably test factual knowledge, and there were ample statistics to demonstrate that the MRCGP multiple choice questionnaire paper could do this reliably. Reliability in this context means that a candidate's mark could be regarded as a true reflection of his or her ability, without being adversely influenced by the different question formats or by the wording within individual questions. It also means that each separate sitting of the exam can be demonstrated to be of comparable difficulty so that candidates of similar ability at different sittings of the exam could be expected to achieve similar scores.

The clinical skills assessment

The clinical skills assessment was devised to assess the practical skills that GPs need, such as clinical examinations and communication.

Some envisaged this component as a form of objective structured clinical examinations (OSCE) in which candidates would visit stations at which they would be expected to demonstrate a specific skill, as commonly used in undergraduate medical exams. This, however, was felt to be too simplistic — it was felt that it was important to test integrative skills, meaning the ability to combine communication skills with clinical skills to gather information and then to use medical knowledge and decision making skills to formulate a management plan. From an early stage it was considered that the best way to do this was using simulated patients. The MRCGP already had a simulated surgery module based on a series of consultations with simulated patients, but this was not felt to be a suitable model for the clinical skills assessment and a working group set about planning the new assessment from scratch.

What they have finally come up with does look remarkably similar to the previous simulated surgery — which is not exactly surprising given that both assessments were designed for the same purpose.

The workplace based assessment

While examinations are a good way of testing knowledge and practical skills, some of the practical skills required are difficult to test in a formal examination setting and are more appropriately assessed in the workplace. It is also difficult to assess attitudinal aspects and professional values in an exam. To get a more holistic assessment of a registrar's competence it was felt that some form of in-training assessment was necessary. This has been present previously with the record of in-training assessment (RITA) during hospital training and the trainer's report in general practice. Although the trainer's report was quite comprehensive and well structured, the workplace based assessment is more rigorous with elements of external assessment and incorporates an objective assessment of consulting skills based on the criteria for the video module of the previous exam.

For the workplace based assessment the GP trainer collects evidence relating to the registrar's performance throughout their training. Much of this will be recorded by the trainer, directly observing and recording the registrar's performance and progress, but there are several specific tools used to record and evaluate this:

- Case-based discussion (CBD), which is a semi-structured interview based on cases
- The consultation observation tool (COT), which is an objective assessment of consulting skills using a video of consultations
- Multi-source feedback (MSF) via questionnaires from colleagues
- Patient satisfaction questionnaires (PSQ)

Progress throughout the workplace based assesment is recorded in the *e*Portfolio, which is an electronic learning log used both as an educational tool and to record successful completion of the main elements (See chapter 4 for more information on the *e*Portfolio).

What happens if I fail?

First of all it is important to say that there is no reason you should fail! To get into training for general practice in the first place you have gone through a fairly rigorous assessment which in fact looks at much the same competencies as *n*MRCGP. The standard of training in general practice is also very high so provided you make the most of your training and prepare yourself well for the assessment you should not have too much difficulty.

The problem facing trainees is that if they have not successfully completed all the modules by the time they finish their training and they have nowhere to go. They cannot enter General Practice as they are not qualified and it is no longer easy to return to hospital for the odd six month job as a stop-gap while they retake modules they have failed. Any trainee who has not passed all the modules will be considered by a Deanery Annual Review of Competency Progression Panel. As long as the Panel considers that the trainee has a good chance of passing with further training it will generally allow an extended period of training, subject to funding being available. To date Deaneries have been able to provide this for the vast majority of trainees.

Most trainees are likely to attempt the applied knowledge test relatively early in speciality trainee level (ST3) or even in speciality trainee level 2 (ST2) so that there are opportunities to attempt it again. There are some arguments against sitting it during speciality training 2, and these will be discussed in Chapter 3.

The clinical skills assessment is more problematic as there are less opportunities to sit this, and sitting it early may significantly increase the risk of failing. Again the reasons for this will be discussed in the relevant chapter.

The workplace based assessment is probably seen as the module least likely to be failed, although it will undoubtedly cause some trainees difficulty. The nature of the workplace based assessment however should mean that difficulties can be identified early and addressed with the trainer.

Ultimately however any additional training period is likely to be limited to six months in general — the old days when doctors could carry on in limbo doing hospital jobs until they passed their exams are gone. If you have not passed all the modules by the end of extended training it is unlikely you will be able to continue on to a career in general practice. Therefore, prepare yourself well and do not waste opportunities.

DH (2001) *Postgraduate Medical Education and Training.* Department of Health, London

The RCGP curriculum

Essentially, the RCGP curriculum sets out what you need to learn throughout GP training. It aims to cover all the areas described in *Good Medical Practice* (General Medical Council [GMC], 2006). The curriculum is divided into six separate domains of competence, and within each of these domains the authors have defined a series of learning outcomes. The six domains are as follows:

- Primary care management
- Person-centred care
- Specific problem-solving skills
- A comprehensive approach
- Community orientation
- A holistic approach.

You can see that although these domains include the factual knowledge required to be a GP, many of them refer more to skills and attitudes. This chapter may seem a bit unnecessary, but it is important as it defines everything you need to know to pass the exam, and throughout the sections of the book describing the various parts of the exam I will refer back to the domains and some of the learning outcomes. The following sections will describe the domains but do not give comprehensive details or listings of all the learning outcomes related to each as these can be downloaded easily from the RCGP website (See Resources section at the end of the book).

As you read through the domains you may think that there is significant overlap between them, and you would be right as there certainly is overlap. Do not be put off by this and do not be put off by the complexity of the curriculum — it is recommended that you read through the College's *Curriculum Guide for Learners and Teachers* (downloadable from the College website), but do not try to memorise it. The whole curriculum is long and detailed and is only really useful to you as reference material rather than as primary reading material. It defines the scope of what the examination sets out to assess you on but is not necessarily terribly useful to you as revision material. In many ways the Curriculum is more useful to GP trainers and programme directors than to trainees since it can be used to plan your educational programmes to ensure coverage of all areas. It is also useful for those setting questions in the exams to ensure they 'sample' from across the curriculum — they clearly cannot ask you everything in the exam so they choose a selection of questions that provides the broadest coverage possible of what is a vast curriculum.

Primary care management

This domain is about the way in which GPs have to be able to deal with anything presented to them. There is generally no filtering before a patient sees a GP and the problem can be from any area within medicine.

The way in which a GP interfaces with the health service is also important, making effective use of services provided by other professionals both within the practice and in secondary care. A GP has to balance doing his best for an individual patient whilst managing resources fairly and effectively. This means the GP needs to have the medical knowledge to deal with acute and chronic conditions, prevent them, palliative care and medical emergencies. To effectively manage these conditions will require communication, clinical examination and therapeutic skills as well as the ability to prioritise. A GP also has to understand how primary care and the wider NHS is organised and needs to be able to work in a team and demonstrate leadership. Use of information technology and an understanding of audit are also important.

This domain describes the concept of patient advocacy, which means communicating with each person as an equal and representing his/her interests with respect to the NHS and other organisation (for example employers, and the Department for Work and Pensions). This must of course be tempered with equality and distributive justice.

The learning outcomes for this domain are knowledge and skill based. You should have sufficient knowledge of the range of illnesses encountered in primary care, as well as understanding of the structure and organisation of the NHS. You should also have organisational, clinical and communication skills, as well as effective teamwork both within the practice and in the interface with secondary care.

Learning points: primary care management

Medical knowledge
IT and audit
Communication
Ability to prioritise
Organisational knowledge
Team-working

Person-centred care

The curriculum describes the following three principles:

- Committing to the person rather than to a particular body of knowledge
- Seeking to understand the context of the illness
- Attaching importance to the subjective aspects of medicine.

This domain is about treating the person rather than the illness, making sure that you fully appreciate the patient's perspective on the problem and incorporates his/her preferences and expectations into any management plan. It does not of course mean simply doing what the patient wants since this may not actually be in the patient's best interests, or there may be issues relating to limited resources, including your time. It does however mean that you should be able to deal with these issues in a way that maintains a good relationship with the patient.

Continuity of care is also key to this domain, maintaining a long-term relationship with a patient, acting in partnership and making shared decisions rather than being paternalistic and making decisions on the patient's behalf.

While knowledge does feature in the learning outcomes for this domain, the emphasis is more on attitude and the communication skills required to fully explore the patient's agenda and integrate the patient's ideas, concerns and expectations into a management plan. It can be helpful to consider consultation models in this domain. The most obviously applicable is that commonly known as *Pendleton*, described in the book *The Consultation – An Approach to Teaching and Learning* and which also discusses the importance of establishing the patient's ideas, concerns and expectations (Pendleton et al, 1984). This has had a profound influence on the development of assessment of communication skills in the MRCGP exam.

In his book *The Inner Consultation*, Neighbour (2004) describes 'connecting', that is, establishing a relationship and rapport with the patient, followed by 'summarising' where the doctor presents his understanding of the patient's problem back to him to check that he has understood the patient correctly. He finally describes 'handing over', which includes explaining the diagnosis and negotiating a mutually acceptable management plan. Contrast this approach with the traditional paternalistic approach where the doctor interrogates the patient, makes a diagnosis and then instructs the patient as to the course of action.

Learning points: person-centred care

Attitude and communication
Exploring the patient's agenda
Care management and planning
Consultation models

Specific problem-solving skills

When we learn to consult patients as medical students and junior doctors we use a systematic approach using a series of questions to cover the whole of a patient's past medical history and all of their clinical systems. This then leads into what is generally referred to as a specialist approach where more detailed examinations and investigations are used to narrow down the problem and reduce uncertainty by systematically excluding conditions.

However this approach does not work in general practice, and the reason why this approach does not work is not only to do with the fact that we do not have the time in a general practice consultation to use it.

In general practice we need to adopt a more problem-based approach where we attempt to focus down very quickly on the patient's problem, using our knowledge of the prevalence of conditions to direct and focus our history-taking and examination. We make decisions based on probability and must accept a degree of uncertainty, often using time to clarify the problem. We analyse and attempt to reduce risks whilst recognising that we cannot completely exclude them, and we must always recognise the need to act urgently where required. This is known as a *generalist approach*.

Generally speaking, a GP will not take a full systematic history but will instead start to consider the possible diagnosis very early on in the consultation and allow this to guide further questioning. Each part of the history will then either add weight or cast doubt on the diagnosis as the consultation proceeds and the probabilities of the differential diagnoses are weighed up.

Apart from saving time, the advantages of a generalist approach includes protecting patients from unnecessary and sometimes unpleasant investigations, as well as the consequent saving of resources. There is also the issue of anxiety — doing more investigations has paradoxically been shown to make patients *more* rather than less worried about the possibility of serious illnesses, even when the investigations turn out to be normal.

The learning outcomes for this domain include knowledge of the incidence and prevalence of diseases and the application of this to an individual patient's social and family context. Knowledge of investigations and treatments available and of their usefulness, as well as their cost, is also important.

The skills required are those needed to gather the appropriate information by taking a history and examining the patient, being able to use the information gained, applying clinical reasoning and making sensible decisions. They also include the skills required to recognise when it is OK to watch and wait, and when it is important to act promptly.

Learning points: specific problem-solving skills

Knowledge of incidence and prevalence of conditions
Knowledge of investigations and costs
History-taking and data gathering
Applying clinical reasoning
Decision-making

A comprehensive approach

Patients rarely present with single isolated problems, and this domain is about managing multiple problems, managing problems within the patient's psycho-social context and integrating preventive medicine and health promotion into the consultation. As a GP you must also provide ongoing care for chronic conditions and in the rehabilitation phase of illnesses.

Learning outcomes for this domain include knowledge of the concept of health and wellbeing, health promotion and of the complexity of problems in general practice.

The skills of managing multiple morbidities and being able to promote health both within the individual consultation and more broadly are also important.

Learning points: a comprehensive approach

Knowledge of health and wellbeing
Health promotion

Community orientation

GPs work within a defined community and it is important to understand the socioeconomic and health features of that community. This domain describes the need to reconcile the needs of the individual patient with those of the community, matched up with the resources available.

The learning outcomes associated with this domain are largely knowledge based — an understanding of the socioeconomic features of the local community and understanding the way they influence health. These factors include poverty, ethnicity, rurality and the area's industrial/commercial history. You should also know the local variations within the healthcare and social services in the area, as well as understanding the roles of other professionals working locally but bearing in mind that since the *n*MRCGP caters for trainees from across the four nations within the UK the questions, either in the AKT or the CSA, must be 'generic' and applicable equally across the board.

Learning points: community orientation

Understanding of socioeconomic features
Understanding and knowledge of local community
Knowledge of local variations in healthcare other social services
Understanding of the role of other local healthcare professionals

---

A holistic approach

The concept of *holism* is an important one to general practice, particularly in the UK where continuing care in long-term relationships with patients is a key feature. Holism means treating the whole patient and considering other issues rather than the purely medical. For example, the person's values which might be based on their culture, ethnicity, religion and the way their family structure influences them. Holism also implies a broader view of interventions, combining psychological, physical and sometimes complementary therapies with the traditional pharmacological ones.

The integration of the physical, psychological and social components of health problems has been well demonstrated to be related to longer consultations and to better continuity of care (Freeman et al, 2002). It is perhaps difficult to reconcile this with modern general practice where continuity is decreasing and quality of care tends to be measured by how quickly a patient can get an appointment than the length of the consultation.

Learning outcomes for this domain include knowledge of holism and how a person's social and psychological circumstances impinge on health as well as knowledge of the patient's cultural background and beliefs. Skill is required to integrate this knowledge into the care of the patient, and attitude aspects such as tolerance and understanding of a patient's beliefs and values are important.

Learning points: a holistic approach

Knowledge of psychological, physical and complementary therapies
Understanding of holism
Tolerance of patient's beliefs and values

Freeman G, Horder J, Howle J, et al (2002) Evolving general practice consultation in Britain: issues of length and context. *BMJ* 324: 880–82

GMC (2006) *Good Medical Practice*. General Medical Council, London

Neighbour R, et al (2004) *The Inner Consultation: How to Develop an Effective and Intuitive Consulting Style*. Radcliffe Publishing, London

Pendleton D, et al (1984) *The Consultation — An Approach to Teaching and Learning*. Oxford University Press, Oxford

Resources

General Medical Council: www.gmc-uk.org
Royal College of General Practitioners: www.rcgp.org

The applied knowledge test

As is obvious from its name, the applied knowledge test is a test of knowledge. What the word 'applied' adds is the explicit statement that it is not simply a test of the simpler 'building blocks' of knowledge you might have, but that the exam tests how you might apply your knowledge to general practice. The knowledge you need is very specific to general practice, rather than just theoretical medical knowledge. For example, rather than simply asking about heart failure, a question might ask about a specific patient, giving a clinical scenario with information about age, sex, specific investigation results and treatment the patient is already on.

The knowledge tested is that required by a working GP in the UK, so it encompasses all the basic knowledge gained throughout medical training but very definitely seeks to test up-to-date evidence-based medicine, therapeutics and current nationally accepted guidelines.

It is impossible to test that a candidate knows everything he/she might need to know as a GP in a single examination, therefore the examiners use sampling, that is dividing the curriculum up into logical areas and asking questions from each area. To make sure that the questions asked adequately represent the breadth of the curriculum requires an adequate sample of questions from each curriculum area, and the more questions the examiners ask the more confident they can be that they have adequately covered the curriculum. There is a limit of course to how many questions they can reasonably ask in a single examination session, so the compromise is reached with a three hour 'paper' and 200 questions.

2.1 Exam format and logistics

The previous MRCGP multiple choice questionnaire was always computer marked, but for the applied knowledge test the College is taking this a step further by making the entire test computer-based.

Each candidate sits the test at a computer station, selecting the correct answers with mouse-clicks instead of the traditional method of shading lozenges with a pencil on a piece of paper. This has several implications for both the College and you as the candidate. For the candidate it removes the potential for errors shading lozenges (they had to be shaded in accurately and there was a risk of shading a lozenge in the wrong row). For the College the most obvious benefit is that the answers can be directly entered into a database thereby removing the risk of misreading the answer sheet.

There are, however, deeper implications than this. Logistically there is a problem being able to provide sufficient computer stations for the 3,000 or more candidates per year. This is solved by using Pearson Vue, best known to most as the company who run the centres at which the UK driving theory test is held. The applied knowledge test is held at Pearson Vue's 147 test centres across the UK, three days per year. Places are allocated on a first come first served basis, so an early application is recommended if you want to sit it at the centre of your choice.

Despite the shift in delivery method, the examination will be essentially the same as the previous MRCGP multiple choice questionnaire in terms of length of the exam, number of questions, question format and the areas covered. The College has significantly increased its bank of questions, allowing different questions to be used each time to reduce the impact of candidates memorising questions and passing them on to colleagues. This, along with high levels of security, means that you are unlikely to encounter 'genuine' applied knowledge test questions either in books, on courses or on websites.

2.2 When to sit the applied knowledge test

It is important to choose the best time to sit the exam; sit it too soon and you run an increased risk of failure as you may not have gained the requisite knowledge. Clearly a candidate is likely to perform best at the end of training, but a failure then may leave no time to re-sit and thus may delay qualification as a GP.

The College recommends that candidates sit the applied knowledge test in the third year of training, ST3, but which sitting to attempt must be an individual decision for each registrar based on confidence in his/her own level of preparation and with some input from the trainer. Although much (but not all) of the clinical medicine will have been learnt before the year in general practice, it is likely that most of the critical appraisal and administration questions will require knowledge gained in general practice. Bear in mind that even material learned while in secondary care may well need to be reconsidered in a general practice context.

The pass rate for ST3 candidates sitting the applied knowledge test for the first time has generally been around 88%, but it is likely to be lower than this. ST2 candidates who have little or no experience of general practice will do relatively poorly on the questions relating to primary care administration.

In theory you are allowed to re-sit the applied knowledge test as many times as you like but of course in reality you need to pass it within your training scheme — if you have not completed it by the end of your training (including any extension granted by your Deanery) then you would still be able to re-sit the applied knowledge test if required.

2.3 Question formats

The applied knowledge test uses several different question formats. The traditional format for medical multiple choice questions was the true/false type where there was typically a description of a question area followed by five different statements each of which were either true or false. This naturally meant that there was a roughly 50% chance of guessing any question correctly even with no medical knowledge. To counter this negative marking was introduced, meaning that a correct answer scored plus one mark, a wrong answer scored a minus one mark, with no mark if the question was left unanswered. Negative marking was dropped after it was made clear that it discriminated against less confident candidates as they would leave blank any questions they were unsure of, whereas the more confident candidates would guess them. In any examination the goal is to accurately discriminate between the good candidates and the weaker ones, and reducing the odds of correctly guessing an answer to below 50% increases this discrimination. The College abandoned the multiple true/false format in the early 90s and no questions in this format appear in the applied knowledge test.

The following is the list of questions formats used, although it is entirely possible that new formats could appear at any time:

- Extended matching questions
- Single best answer
- Multiple best answers
- Picture format
- Table/algorithm completion
- Data interpretation
- Seminal trials

During the exam a simple example will be given for each format purely to demonstrate the format. Examples of each format are available on the College's website.

2.3.1 Extended matching questions
In this question format a range of options are provided as answers, and each separate question is a short scenario. You must choose the correct answer from the range of options for each scenario. Each answer carries one mark.

It will be specified that **only one** option is correct. Although you may consider more than one option to be plausible, one will be the single most appropriate answer. This will generally be based on an authoritative source such as the British National Formulary (BNF), a nationally recognised guideline or a piece of important published research.

You can see from the example box that using this format means random guesses would be expected to yield a mark of 12.5%.

Extended matching question

Theme: Management of hypertension

Option list:
        a. Lifestyle advice
        b. Bendroflumethiazide
        c. Atenolol
        d. Lisinopril
        e. Irbesartan
        f. Methyldopa
        g. Nifedipine
        h. Doxazosin

Instruction: For each patient with hypertension select the single most appropriate treatment. Each answer may be used once, more than once, or not at all. Items:

1. A 79-year-old non-diabetic patient with no significant past medical history and repeated blood pressure readings averaging 155/85.

2. A 79-year-old diabetic patient with repeated blood pressure readings averaging 155/85.

3. A 57-year-old Afro-Caribbean man with repeated blood pressure readings averaging 155/85 who is already taking indapamide 2.5mg daily.

2.3.2 Single best answer

The odds are a little better here at 1 in 7, but the question is made more difficult by more than one option appearing plausible. More than one of these treatments has been claimed or shown to be effective in premenstrual syndrome, but recent evidence suggests one to be superior to the others.

2.3.3 Multiple best answers

This is similar to the single best answer format but where you are asked to specify a given number of options. In the example box given, each answer carries one mark, the order in which you choose them does not matter. Although you might think the odds reduce from 1 in 10 to 1 in 9 once you have made your first choice that is only true if you have got the first one right. Note that the question refers very specifically to the published NICE guidelines although even without having read them it is possible to organise the options into some form of order of probability based on your general medical knowledge and experience.

Single best answer

According to current evidence, which treatment provides the greatest benefit in premenstrual syndrome? Select one answer only

a. Fluoxetine
b. Mefenamic acid
c. Norethisterone
d. The combined oral contraceptive pill
e. Evening primrose oil
f. Depo-provera
g. Vitamin B6

Multiple best answer

According to the NICE guidelines for management of feverish illness in children, which THREE of the following features are NOT classified within the RED category:

Option List:

a. Non-blanching rash
b. Dry mucous membrane
c. Appears ill to a healthcare professional
d. Oxygen saturation ≤95% in air
e. Weak, high pitched or continuous cry
f. Grunting
g. Respiratory rate more than 40 breaths/minute and age more than 12 months
h. Bile-stained vomiting
i. Focal neurological signs
j. Age 0–3 months, temperature more than 38°C

2.3.4 Table/algorithm completion

In this more graphical question format you are provided with a table or an algorithm (a chart usually depicting a clinical care pathway) where some of the text has been removed. You need to select the appropriate option for each space from a list. See example box on the next page. Again in this case the odds of guessing are low, at 1 in 8 for each item, although some are easily excluded. We will discuss strategies for answering questions in a later section.

Table/algorithm completion

The UK Resuscitation Council Automated external defibrillator resuscitation (AED) algorithm

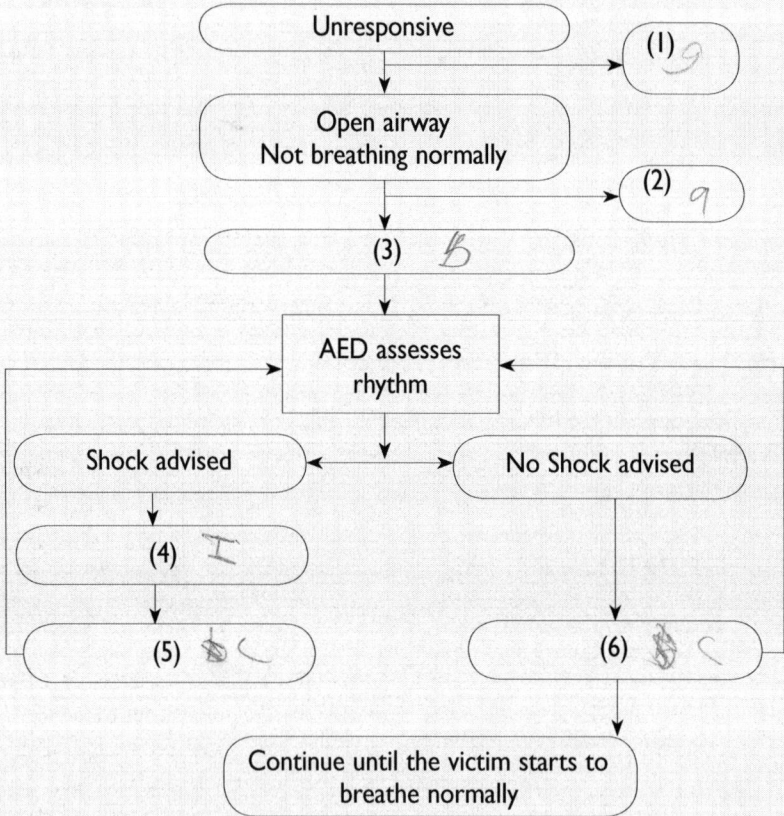

Unresponsive → (1) *g*

↓

Open airway
Not breathing normally → (2) *q*

↓

(3) *b*

↓

AED assesses rhythm

Shock advised ← → No Shock advised

Shock advised
↓
(4) *I*
↓
(5) *(handwritten)*

No Shock advised
↓
(6) *(handwritten)*

↓

Continue until the victim starts to breathe normally

For each of the numbered gaps select **ONE** option from the list below. Each option may be used once, more than once, or not at all. Select **ONE** option only.

a. Check for pulse
b. CPR 30:2 until AED is attached
c. Immediately resume CPR 30:2 for 2 minutes
d. Administer oral aspirin
e. Send or go for AED. Call 999
f. 1 shock 150-360J biphasic or 360J monophasic
g. Call for help
h. Insert oral airway

2.3.5 Data interpretation

In this format the examiners can assess your ability to understand various presentations of statistical data. This may be in the form of a series of numbers, data table, or any of the graphical presentations of data such as graphs, bar charts, Forest plots, and so on. It is clear here that you must have a good understanding of the statistical terms referred to — if you do the questions are quite easy. We will discuss the terms and graphical presentation methods you need to know about in a later section. Consider the example overleaf. This format of question can be quite difficult to grasp, especially in the stress of an exam, so perhaps it will be helpful to go through this example in a little more detail.

The table overleaf shows data from an imaginary trial of a screening test for carcinoma of the prostate. Let us first of all just clarify what the rows and column in the table mean. The top row shows the number of patients who had a positive test with the total on the far right (5). The row below shows those who had a negative test again with the total on the far right (95), thus the total number in this trial was 100, which is shown in the bottom right cell. The numbers are subdivided into two columns depending on whether the patients actually did have the disease or not, with totals on the bottom row.

The right hand column tells you that of these 100 patients 5 had a positive test while the remaining 95 were negative. The bottom row tells you that of the 100 patients 6 were known to have the disease while the remaining 94 did not. The left column tells you that of these 6 patients with the disease, 4 had a positive test while the other two tested negative. The middle column tells you that 1 patient who did not have the disease had a positive test, while the remaining 93 disease-free patients tested negative.

Moving on to the question items, the first one, the sensitivity of the test, refers to the proportion of true positives that are correctly identified by the test. In this example we can see that there were 6 true positives of whom 4 were correctly identified. Therefore the answer is 4/6 which is option '*m*'.

Item two asks for the specificity of the test which refers to the proportion of true negatives that are correctly identified by the test. Here we have 94 true negatives of whom 93 correctly had a negative test so the answer is 93/94 which is option '*p*'.

Item three asks for the positive predictive value. This is the reliability with which a positive test correctly identifies a patient with the disease. In this example there were 5 positive tests of whom 4 actually had the disease, so the positive predictive value is 4/5 which is option '*a*'.

The negative predictive value in item four refers to the reliability with which a negative test identifies a patient who does not have the disease. Here there were 95 patients who tested negative of whom 93 were actually disease-free, giving a negative predictive value of 93/95.

Item five asks for the prevalence of the disease in the study population. This is simply the number who did have the disease as a proportion of the total, in this case 6 out of 100 which is option '*f*'.

Data interpretation

The following data is from a trial of a new screening test for carcinoma of the prostate. The numbers represent the number of patients in the trial for each category

	Disease	No Disease	Total
Positive test	4	1	5
Negative test	2	93	95
Total	6	94	100

Option list: The numbers below reflect the numbers from the table as fractions

a. 4/5
b. 1/5
c. 2/95
d. 93/95
e. 2/93
f. 6/100
g. 6/94
h. 93/100

i. 94/100
j. 95/100
k. 5/95
l. 5/100
m. 4/6
n. 2/6
o. 1/94
p. 93/94
q. none of these

For each of the following items select the most appropriate answer from the options list above.

Items:

1. The sensitivity of the test M
2. The specificity of the test P
3. The positive predictive value of the test a 4/5
4. The negative predictive value of the test d 93/95
5. The prevalence of the disease among the sample of the trial 6/100

Two specific formats for presenting statistical data are worth mentioning as they have both come up as applied knowledge test questions — the **forest plot** and the **funnel plot**. A forest plot (also sometimes known as a '*blobbogram*' or '*box and whisker*' plot) is a way of graphically displaying data from multiple trials in a meta-analysis. A further example is currently given within the applied knowledge test Power Point presentation downloadable from the College website.) The x-axis represents the size of the treatment effect (sometimes with a logarithmic scale) and each trial is represented as a row in the plot up the y-axis. Underneath in the bottom row will be a summation of the data from all the trials. The salient features of a forest plot are listed below:

* A square (the blob or box) representing the result for each trial. The position of the square represents the mean result from that trial and the size of it represents the size of the study so a large square means it was a large study and vice versa
* A horizontal line through each square representing the 95% confidence intervals. This means that, statistically speaking, you can be 95% confident that the actual result of the study lies within the range of this line. Generally speaking larger studies will have shorter lines meaning tighter confidence intervals, smaller studies will have longer ones
* At the side of the chart the actual values for the mean and the confidence intervals will usually be displayed as numbers
* A line of no effect is shown as a vertical line to represent the point at which the trials show no difference between treatment and control groups. The important point about this is that if the confidence interval line for a particular trial crosses the line of no effect that trial is NOT statistically significant
* A diamond at the bottom of the plot representing the summation of the studies. Again the centre of the diamond shows the mean result but this time the 95% confidence intervals are represented by the overall width of the diamond. Because this is the overall meta-analysis and the numbers of patients involved is therefore greater than all the other trials individually the confidence intervals are generally fairly narrow. As with the individual squares, if the diamond crosses the line of no effect this means that the meta-analysis does not show a statistically significant treatment effect.

A funnel plot is another way of graphically representing data from multiple trials in a meta-analysis. Each trial is displayed in a scatter plot with treatment effect on the x (horizontal) axis and study size on the y (vertical) axis. In a perfect world all the studies would show the same treatment effect so all the points would appear in a vertical line stacked on top of each other but this never happens. What generally happens is that there is variation between the studies and smaller studies tend to have more variation than larger ones so they appear at the left and right hand margins of the plot while the larger studies tend to show similar results and appear in the middle. This gives the overall appearance of an inverted cone, or funnel, hence the name.

If the plot does not appear symmetrical this suggests either that for some reason the smaller trials genuinely do give different results (perhaps because the study protocols do not match those of the larger ones — heterogeneity) or that some trials have not been included in the meta-analysis — this is known as publication bias. Publication bias is the phenomenon whereby trials showing a positive (or strongly negative) outcome are more likely to get published in peer reviewed journals than trials showing no difference in outcomes between the treatment group and the controls.

Forest plots are generally more useful and are used far more frequently in journals than funnel plots and as a consequence appear far more frequently in the applied knowledge test. However a funnel plot has appeared in a past sitting of the exam so it is worth being aware of them. Ten minutes revision of these graphical formats in the days before the exam can mean collecting easy marks if they come up.

2.3.6 Seminal trials

This format allows the examiners to test knowledge previously tested in written papers. It allows them to test knowledge of very specific clinical trials, which can include very recent data. For this sort of question you are likely to be asked about any relevant aspects of the methodology and about the results. Do not worry too much about remembering dates, authors, the journal articles were published, etc.

Seminal trial

Regarding the Scandinavian Simvastatin Survival Study
(Lancet 1994; 344: 1383-89)

Which THREE of the following statements are correct:

  a. This study is an example of primary prevention
  b. The follow-up period was over five years
  c. There was no difference in non-cardiovascular deaths
  d. The trial results were published as absolute risk reductions
  e. There was a significant reduction in all-cause mortality in women
  f. The absolute risk reductions for those aged over 65 years were roughly double that for the aged under 65 years
  g. This was a cohort study
  h. The study was a randomised controlled trial
  i. The NNT for mortality was 12

2.4 Question areas

About 80% of the questions in the applied knowledge test are on clinical medicine, 10% on critical appraisal and evidence-based medicine and the remaining 10% on health informatics and administration.

2.4.1 Clinical medicine

The problem with clinical medicine is that as GPs we see undifferentiated problems, and as patients can turn up with *any* problem you might think you need to know *everything*. Clearly that is simply not feasible, so the trick in preparing for the exam is to be selective. Looking through the examiners' comments on the College website can be quite illuminating in considering how the examiners choose the topics for questions. The important thing to remember is that this is an exam about *general practice*, so it is important to know a lot about the things we see frequently, but it is reasonable to expect a lower level of knowledge for the rarer problems. This presents a bit of a dilemma though from a safety point of view — what about the patient who turns up with something rare but with potentially serious consequences? The answer is of course that we need to know enough about the less common but serious problems to be able to spot them when they do present; we must have good self-awareness about the areas in which we are weaker and we need to recognise an ill patient who needs urgent action.

Considering the various areas described in the curriculum can be helpful. They can be divided according to which clinical system they affect:

* Cardiovascular problems
* Digestive problems
* Drug and alcohol problems
* Ear, nose and throat (ENT) and facial problems
* Eye problems
* Metabolic problems
* Neurological problems
* Respiratory problems
* Rheumatology and conditions of the musculoskeletal system (including trauma)
* Skin problems (dermatology).
* Genito-urinary.

The curriculum also discusses these areas in groupings according to age/sex, and a couple of broader clinical areas:

* Healthy people: promoting health and preventing disease
* Genetics in primary care
* Care of acutely ill people

- Care of children and young people
- Care of older adults
- Gender-specific health issues
- Women's health
- Men's health
- Sexual health
- Care of people with cancer and palliative care
- Care of people with mental health problems
- Care of people with learning disabilities.

2.4.2 Critical appraisal and evidence-based medicine

Critical appraisal is the skill of being able to read a piece of material and appraise it from several points of view. Try asking yourself the following questions when appraising material: Is it relevant to me as a GP? Is the methodology appropriate to the aims of the work? Is there any bias? Are the findings significant and are the conclusions appropriate to the findings?

Relevance is important — this can be about how common or important the subject matter is to general practice or it can be about the context of the work, for example studies done in secondary care. It is important to understand the various kind of methodology used in studies. The following is a list of the main methodologies:

Case report or series
A report on a single case or a limited number of cases, generally where something unusual has happened. An example of this would be a report of a patient suffering unexpected side effects from a drug.

Cohort study Prospective
A longitudinal study where a specific group of subjects are followed up over a period of time to observe what happens to them. An example of this would be following up a group of patients with a raised PSA to observe the incidence of prostatic carcinoma. There would usually be a control group (of patients with a normal PSA) for comparison. Note that this methodology is *prospective*.

Case control study Retrospective
This is where individuals with a condition are matched with controls who do not have the condition but who are similar in other ways (e.g. age, sex). An example would be looking at patients with breast cancer and comparing them with similar controls to identify potential risk factors. Note that this methodology is *retrospective*. See below for further discussion of this. Note also that any factors identified are *associations* rather than necessarily being *causes*.

Prospective study
This is a study in which all the study parameters are defined and study population

identified before the intervention is applied or before they are divided into groups and observed longitudinally. This includes all randomised trials and some cohort studies.

Retrospective study
The study parameters are defined, then the researchers look back at what has already happened to the study population. This includes most case control studies and retrospective cohort studies. While retrospective studies have the advantage that they can often be done quickly (since all the data is generally already available) the disadvantage is that there is potentially more risk of bias or confounding.

Uncontrolled trial
Where a group of subjects are subjected to an intervention (such as a drug treatment) and followed up to observe the effect. A drawback with this methodology is that any observed improvements (or deteriorations) may have arisen anyway and may not necessarily be as a result of the intervention.

Randomised control trial gold standard pr CDM
This is the better method of investigating the effects of an intervention. The subjects are allocated at random to receive either the intervention or to be controls. The control group may receive no intervention, a placebo or a different form of intervention (for instance where a new drug is compared with the current usual therapy for a condition).

Systematic review
This is a form of review where the researcher looks for all relevant research articles on a subject and analyses them to produce a summary.

Meta-analysis ✕ gold standard for CDM
This is similar to a systematic review but the researcher actually combines the raw data gathered in the original research articles and combines it all to produce a single large dataset. This is useful when studies show very small effects or where results of different studies are conflicting, often as a result of studies being small and lacking power. The randomised controlled trial and the meta-analysis are considered the gold standard for evidence-based medicine.

Qualitative research
The methodologies described above are mostly quantitative — that is they produce numbers which can be analysed statistically. Some research subjects are not suitable to this approach however, for example where the researchers are investigating peoples' views on a subject, or investigating the effect an illness. Typically they involve questionnaires and interviews to generate their information.

There are several types of *bias* that can afflict clinical papers.

- **Selection bias** is where the people being studied are in some way selected and not necessarily representative of the general population. Examples include studies on students, prisoners, or volunteers, or where certain groups (for example the elderly) are excluded from a study.
- **Information bias** is caused by data gathering having a subjective element
- **Observer bias** is a form of information bias where measurements taken may not be consistent depending on who takes them. **Inter-observer bias** would be, for example, where different clinicians taking the same measurement on the same patient would obtain different values. **Intra-observer** bias is where the same clinician obtains different values, for example, checking the same patient's blood pressure several times within a few minutes and recording different readings.
- **Recall bias** is another source of information bias where subjects are asked to recall what has happened. For example, asking patients how long they waited for their doctor to arrive when they called with chest pain.
- **Confounding bias** is where factors other than the ones being studied may account for an observed effect. For example, the finding that beer drinkers are more likely to suffer from lung cancer than non-beer drinkers. The confounding factor here of course is that it is likely the beer drinkers are more likely to be smokers than the non-beer drinkers.

Statistics causes many registrars a headache but in reality you probably do not need to know as much as you think you might. One of the most common problems encountered is that most statistical textbooks, even the fairly basic ones, provide more depth than is needed, which causes confusion. It is easy to read a chapter and think you have understood it only to find 10 minutes later that you cannot remember it. The solution here is to limit your learning to the basics. Here is my list of the terms and concepts you should try to make sure you understand:

- Normal distribution and what the terms median and mode mean
- Probability, including p values and confidence intervals
- Correlation, including what a *chi-squared test* is for
- Sensitivity, specificity, positive and negative predictive values
- Relative and absolute risk reduction, including the ability to calculate numbers needed to treat (NNT) from some simple figures
- Odds ratios.

Make sure you are aware of the common ways of presenting statistical data, such as graphs showing positive or negative correlation, and forest plots. There is an excellent *BMJ* article which explains them fully (Lewis and Clarke, 2001). In the old style MRCGP knowledge of the points above were often asked in the critical reading questions within the written paper. Look through the past papers on the College website to see some example of statistic depth required for the exam.

This section has just been a short summary of research methodologies and critical appraisal, and a more detailed discussion is beyond the scope of this book. There are plenty of resources for learning about critical appraisal including *How to Read a Paper* by Greenhalgh, originally written as a series of articles for the *BMJ* but later published as a book.

The sources used for the evidence-based medicine questions will be discussed in a later section.

2.5 Health informatics and administration

Modern general practice is heavily dependent on information technology. This requires an understanding of computers, clinical coding, searching data and data management. The College recommends that registrars should have reached the standard of the European Computer Driving Licence (ECDL) by the end of their GP training programme. Make sure you know about this (See the Resources section at the end of this chapter).

The term *information governance* describes the management of confidentiality in an electronic world. It is important that you have an awareness of the legislation covering this in the UK — you do not need to know the law in depth but you need to be aware of the implications for the GP in his/her daily work. Find out who the Caldicott Guardian is in your practice and speak to them about what their role entails. Make sure you understand the issues relating to use of patient records for reports to third parties such as insurance companies, etc. and that you understand the Data Protection Act 1998.

You can do most of the revision on health informatics and administration you need for the *n*MRCGP from your computer. Make sure you understand how to make the most of it, consider how and why you use each internet-based tool. Other questions in this section relate to aspects of general practice administration. The following lists some of the ones you need to know about:

- Sickness certification
- Fitness to drive guidelines
- Employment law
- Health and safety at work
- Control of Substances Hazardous to Health (CoSHH) legislation
- The General Medical Services contract and Quality and Outcomes (QOF) Framework

These will not be detailed in this book as it is very easy to source the information you need from the internet.

2.6 How to prepare for the paper

The sure way to pass the applied knowledge test is to know everything there is to know in the curriculum areas. However this is not possible, and the reason you are reading this book is to improve your chances of passing the exam with the minimal expenditure of time and effort.

There are two ways a book like this can help you — firstly by giving guidance on how to make the best use of your revision time and secondly by giving advice on examination technique. This section will deal with the former, while examination technique will be covered in the last section in this chapter.

There is also the issue of how to divide your revision time between the different areas of the paper. Clinical medicine accounts for 80% of the questions so it might seem intuitive to concentrate on this. The problem with this approach is that the area is so vast it requires a huge amount of work to revise enough to make a difference. The mean score in this area is usually around 75%, i.e. most candidates do relatively well. Improving in an area you are already doing well in requires more effort than an area where you are performing poorly as there are more knowledge gaps to fill. The mean score in the area of evidence interpretation is about 72% but clearly it is a much more tightly defined area with a much greater probability that anything new you learn might actually come up in the exam. The same applies to the organisational questions — a few hours revision in this area can cover a much bigger proportion of the curriculum. In addition the mean score in this area has usually been below 60% so it is the area in which the average candidate has the most scope to improve.

2.6.1 Key topics

Adult education should be specific to the learner, identifying their needs and meeting them in ways that suit their learning style. However, no doubt at the start of your practice year your trainer will have identified some key basics that you would need to cover.

The same principle applies to the applied knowledge test; there are some topics that it is worth listing and revising systematically as they are very likely to come up in the exam. The list below is focused on those topics that are relatively easy to revise as they are fairly finite topics and they have very specific, definitive resources that you can access easily:

- Guidelines (e.g. NICE/SIGN)
- National Service Frameworks
- Fitness to drive guidance
- Drug interactions
- *BNF* guidance on prescribing
- *Drug and Therapeutics Bulletin*
- Key legislation
- Key *BMJ* articles

Guidelines

The National Institute for Clinical Effectiveness (NICE) and the Scottish Intercollegiate Guidelines Network (SIGN) are bodies which regularly publish nationally accepted guidelines. Although both organisations do publish paper copies of their work, they both have up-to-date, well maintained websites with easy access to all their guidance. Have a good look at both sites and look through the guidelines published within the last couple of years. Some will have little or no relevance to general practice, so exercise judgement as to which ones you think it is worth spending some time on.

As discussed earlier concentrate on both the topics that you commonly deal with as a GP and those that are less common but important to get right. It is worth writing a summary of each and keeping these together so you can read through your summary again. If you have friends locally who are also preparing for the exam you can pool efforts by allocating the various guidelines among yourselves and sharing the summaries you produce. Actually discussing them in a group session makes it more likely you will remember the information.

In addition there are a few key guidelines published by other bodies, particularly the medical Royal Colleges. These include the British Thoracic Society guidelines for asthma in adults and children and the British Hypertension Society guidelines (see resources section).

National Service Frameworks

These are strategies published by the Department of Health to set standards and suggest strategies for providers of healthcare. There are summaries of each on the NHS and Department of Health websites and you should be aware of those published so far. These currently include:

- Cancer
- Children
- Chronic obstructive pulmonary disease
- Coronary heart disease
- Diabetes
- Long-term conditions
- Mental health
- Older people
- Renal services

Learning the detail of them all would be a daunting task but whenever new ones are published they become prime material for applied knowledge test questions.

Fitness to drive

Guidance is published by the Driver and Vehicle Licensing Agency (DVLA) and while there will probably be a paper copy in your practice, the most recent guidance can be downloaded from the DVLA website. Again there is a bit too much here to learn it all but make sure you know the areas that are likely to crop up in your work as a GP. These include myocardial infarction and angina, epilepsy and other causes of loss of consciousness, transient ischaemic attack and stroke.

Drug interactions
These have always been a regular feature in the MRCGP multiple choice questionnaire and it seems likely they will remain so in the applied knowledge test. They have always been an important topic but current chronic disease management encourages polypharmacy like never before, thereby making interactions more important than ever. Again you cannot really just revise the whole *British National Formulary* section on interactions so you must be selective. The general principle remains that you must focus on the common ones and on those that are potentially serious. Make sure you read up on interactions with warfarin, oral contraceptives and anticonvulsants particularly. A related area is that of drugs that are particularly likely to cause side-effects or which require specific monitoring such as the disease modifying anti-rheumatic drugs.

The British National Formulary
In addition to looking up specific items it is well worth spending an hour or two reading through the sections containing guidance on prescribing at the front of the book. This includes guidance on writing prescriptions writing, emergency supply of medicines, controlled drugs, adverse reactions, prescribing for children, the elderly, palliative care and emergency treatment of poisoning. Each section also has specific prescribing advice although this may be best read when you look up individual drugs.

Drug and Therapeutics Bulletin
This is now published by the BMJ Group, is independent of government and the NHS, and is highly respected as an authoritative source of prescribing information. It is published fortnightly, and it is well worth looking through the last 12 to 18 months' issues to identify any topics you think look important. It is available online but you will need either a BMA subscription or an Athens username and password to access it. As a GP registrar you should be able to have access, so ask your trainer about it.

Key legislation
There are aspects of legislation that are important and worth summarising for revision. As mentioned already make sure you know about the Data Protection Act, Access to Medical Records Act, Health and Safety at Work, COSHH and Advance Directives.

The British Medical Journal
Is a major source of information for the nMRCGP. Lots of questions are based on *BMJ* articles, particularly from the educational ABC series and themed issues. The *BMJ* website organises these nicely for you. As previously mentioned the online *BMJ* also gives you access to the excellent series of articles on critical reading.

2.6.2 Identifying educational needs
Identifying your educational needs is of great importance when the amount of potential material as so vast and your time is limited.

The first opportunity we will discuss is what is called *experiential learning* which is basically learning by experiences. The trouble is that you do not learn purely from experience, but the experience of seeing patients and working in a primary care team provides you with daily prompts of the things you do not know so well as you should. Make sure you switch your autopilot off and think about everything you do. Hopefully as a registrar you have enough breathing space to be able to reflect between consultations. Keep a notebook with you and jot down any knowledge gaps you spot during the working day.

The term *PUNS and DENs* was coined in the early 90s by Richard Eve, a GP tutor who described the process of identifying when you had encountered a knowledge gap (**P**atient's **U**nmet **N**eed) and by jotting it down and reflecting upon it later to convert it into a focused educational need (**D**octor's **E**ducational **N**eed) (Eve, 2003). For every diagnosis think of the differential — are you confident of the aetiology of the illness, any diagnostic criteria and appropriate investigations? Are there any guidelines for referral or management?

Think about every prescription. Doctors often prescribe a drug because it is what they are comfortable with, often because it was a consultant's 'favourite' drug during the early formative months in their medical career. While the drug might well be the correct choice we should always be consciously aware of why we are prescribing it, what the benefits of the individual drug are and of the potential risks of prescribing it.

Another opportunity for identifying learning needs is in your general reading and keeping up-to-date with current journals. Doctors have a habit of sticking to what they know, but you need to learn the habit of identifying topics you think you do not know enough about.

Scan the *BMJ* weekly, again being selective to identify articles of relevance to you. Do not just read the editorials, research articles and the ABC series; the news pages often have reports on important work published elsewhere such as the *New England Journal of Medicine* and the *Lancet*. Any obvious important papers are likely to be discussed in the editorial and are likely to be discussed in the weekly magazines such as *Pulse* and *GP*. The letters section of the *BMJ* is often interesting as it contains other readers comments on articles pointing out flaws or other work which conflicts with the authors conclusions, and the online journal allows for the fairly interactive *rapid responses* which make the debate much more real-time.

2.6.3 Meeting educational needs

Meeting your educational needs is actually the easy bit, it just requires the discipline and commitment. Accessing the resources you need has never been easier — long gone are the days of trawling through Index Medicus in the local medical library. When it comes to looking up a topic you have identified as a learning need, there are a few key resources. The vast majority of questions devised for the applied knowledge test will be based on information from a handful of sources:

*   The *British Medical Journal*
*   *Clinical Evidence*
*   The *British National Formulary* and other resources already discussed above.

We have already discussed the *BMJ*, but there are a couple of other points to make about using it to look up a topic. You can simply use the website search facility but the problem then is that quite often it returns too many results. Check to see if what you are interested in has been the subject of a themed issue, an ABC series or an *Education and Debate* article. The journal also has a section of collected resources where articles are grouped according to subject area (for example diabetes, coronary heart disease), which can make life much easier.

Clinical Evidence is another publication by the *BMJ* group and appears in a book about the same size as the BNF as well as on the website. The advantage of the website is that it is always up to date and it is searchable. You should be able to gain full access to the website via your NHS intranet connection; it is available by subscription otherwise. *Clinical Evidence* is the definitive resource for many of the clinical questions and takes the form of systematic reviews of the topics covered. It is not completely comprehensive and a lot of its content is not directly relevant to GPs, so use it to look things up rather than as a book to browse.

Bandolier is another useful resource, published by the Oxford Centre for Evidence Based Medicine. Again the website is easy to use with a good search facility.

GP Notebook is a popular resource for both doctors and patients. It is user friendly and is easy to read, but beware that although the information given is referenced it is not a definitive resource. As its name suggests it is really aimed at general practice and most searches deliver highly relevant content. Its ease of use makes it ideal for looking things up quickly between patients, or even with the patient there.

2.6.4 Practice questions

It is always helpful to practice past papers when preparing for a multiple choice examination. However times change and there are reasons why this might not be as helpful as it used to be. In multiple choice question papers of old it was possible to improve your mark purely via examination technique — deducing right or wrong answers from the wording of the question. A huge amount of effort has gone into eliminating this from the applied knowledge test so it is a very pure test of your actual knowledge of the subject area.

There are many books of practice questions for the nMRCGP, and some of these seem to reappearing re-badged as applied knowledge test practice questions which is probably reasonable enough since they are mostly from the same question bank. There are also websites offering practice questions. Authors write these questions generally in one of two ways. The first method is to actually create the questions themselves from scratch which has the disadvantage that the authors do not generally have the expertise of the group of authors who write the genuine questions, nor do they have the psychometric backup and experience required to construct question that are valid and reliable while offering the appropriate degree of difficulty (we will discuss features that affect the degree of difficulty in the next section).

The second method is essentially plagiarising questions by getting candidates to recall questions when they sit the exam. This causes different problems. To avoid copyright infringement authors have to change the wording slightly, which can completely change the integrity of a question. This also gives the College a bit of a headache as it wishes to maintain the integrity of its question bank. This is even more the case now that the applied knowledge test is part of a licensing examination. Of course the examiners know which questions have been compromised so they are likely to be removed from the question bank. Practising these questions does have its usefulness but you are not likely to see any of them in the live exam and indeed a batch of question that became compromised in this was is used as sample practice questions at the start of the applied knowledge test.

So what is the benefit of practice questions? The main benefit is that you get to test your knowledge in the areas that the exam covers and gain experience with the various question formats. You can also get an idea of how quickly or slowly you can answer the questions. To some extent, possibly more so with the questions taken from the exam, you can get an idea of how well you are doing.

2.7 How to maximise your performance on the day

2.7.1 Getting there on time and in the right frame of mind
You have been preparing for months, and finally the big day arrives. It is very important to get it right on the day, so this section will discuss how you can try to ensure that you perform at your best.

First consider the day before. It may sound really obvious but make sure you give yourself a chance by not turning up tired. It is unlikely in this day and age that you will be on call the night before the exam, but try to relax and make sure you get enough sleep. You will not improve your performance by burning the midnight oil reading journals. It might be worth glancing through any revision notes you have made but do not sit reading all evening. Similarly having a big party night probably is not such a good idea. Do something that will relax you and take your mind off the exam; that might mean spending time with family or some friends, going to the cinema, maybe some exercise. Do not spend it with friends who are also doing the exam the next day as the conversation will inevitably focus on the exam and some bright spark will manage to mention all the things you do not think you have revised enough or some important paper you have never heard of.

Make sure you know exactly where you are going and allow enough time to travel. Roads can get very congested and a minor accident tends to cause interminable delays. If you are driving make sure you know where to park. It is tempting to travel with friends, but if you do make sure they are not going to make you late and ensure you agree to leave at a time you are comfortable with. Make a contingency plan in case there is a problem, for example a car not starting. If you are late you will not be allowed into the exam. Another disadvantage of lift-sharing is again the issue of talking about the exam — it inevitably makes you more nervous rather than less. Try to find something else to talk about, for example football, your trainer's latest awful tie, anything rather than the exam.

Pearson Vue will try to ensure the temperature in the exam centre is comfortable but if it is too warm or too cold for you three hours can be a long time so make sure you are dressed comfortably with layers you can add/remove.

When you get to the centre you will need to prove you are who you say you are by producing photo identification so make sure you have read your instructions carefully and can provide the required ID. There will be a quarantine system to prevent candidates sitting the exam in the morning communicating with those sitting in the afternoon. The implications of this are that if you are sitting in the morning you will not be allowed to leave early, and if you are sitting in the afternoon you will not be allowed in if you arrive late.

When you arrive you will not be allowed to take anything into the examination room with you. This includes writing implements, mobile phones or other electronic devices and food/drink. Water will be provided for you and you will be given an erasable note board for jotting notes which will then be retained in the room. You can also jot notes electronically on a scratch-pad facility on the computer.

Using the computer should not be an issue as it is likely you use a computer every day of the week. If you have any problems ask the staff for help as that is what they are there for. You can access a tutorial on the Pearson Vue website and I strongly recommend that you have a go at this at least once before you take the exam.

When you get into the centre you will be able to complete a 10 minute tutorial with sample nMRCGP questions before you start the real exam. Answering the questions is simple, you just click on the button next to your chosen answer, the letter next to it (i.e. A, B, C, etc.) or on the actual text of the answer. You can also choose an option via the appropriate letter on the computer keyboard.

Before you start answering the questions make sure you read the instructions provided. These will include a brief glossary of terms such as *in the majority, in the minority, has been shown, recognised* and *reported*; make sure you understand these and any other instructions before you proceed.

2.7.2 Answering the questions

Make sure you read the questions carefully. Take the questions at face value and trust the examiners as a lot of effort has been put into making the questions as clear, unambiguous and fair as is possible. Do not look for hidden meanings and trick questions as there genuinely aren't any.

There will be a huge range of questions, not only in the areas they are testing, but also in the degree of difficulty. Of course if you know the answer any question is easy, but there will be some questions that will be genuinely difficult and inevitably you will come across some questions where you really have not got a clue. Do not panic, read the question carefully and apply some of the strategies outlined below. Remember that the pass mark is usually around 65% — you can afford to get over 30% of the questions wrong and still pass! There will always be questions that completely stump you, the trick is to not allow them to put you off.

If you read the question and know the answer straight away without even looking through the options just double check to make sure you have read the question correctly and through the options to make sure you are not missing something, then record your answer and move on to the next question. There will be plenty of questions that appear easy and it is sometimes possible to be put off by this, worrying that if it seems easy you must be missing something important.

However for the majority of the questions you will need to apply more thought. Maybe there are a couple of the options that you think might be correct, in which case concentrate on those to see which you think the more likely. Maybe there are a couple of the options that you know are wrong, in which case you can narrow your odds down a bit. Occasionally there are words in the options that can help you, such as *never* or *always* — it is rare in medicine for something to be always or never true. However the examiners know these words give you clues so will try to avoid using them in the questions.

Once you have excluded what you can — if you really are not sure — and what you cannot choose between the remaining options, you will need to guess.

Whatever you do, **do not fail to answer a question**, you really must have a guess or you are wasting a chance of a mark. Be aware that even when you are not sure your guesses are not random, they may be informed by partial recall of something you have read in the past. You have the choice of either leaving the question and coming back to it or committing yourself to a guess straight away.

Deferring your answer has the advantage that when you come back it might appear clearer or you might have remember something useful. If you guess you can still go back and change your answer later if you like.

Do not be disheartened by the questions you do not know, the chances are if you are sitting there thinking a particular question is difficult most of your fellow sufferers will be thinking the same. You know before you go in there that you are never going to get 100%, so give each question your best shot then move on without getting upset about it. Just make sure you attempt each question with a clear head as worrying about the previous question will only impair your performance.

Keep an eye on the time. The computer screen will continuously display the time remaining. Most people have enough time to complete the exam comfortably, but you will not finish as early as you might have in the past with the older format of multiple true/false answers.

Once you have finished check to make sure you have answered all the questions. Some candidates prefer to go through some of the questions they were less sure about again, whilst others prefer to have one first try at them and not go back. This is down to your own personality, but generally speaking going back changing answers is not a good idea unless you really have remembered something new as there is a risk you change a correct guess into a wrong guess, as well as vice-versa.

If you want to leave a question until later you can as it is easy enough to revisit your unanswered questions at the end of the exam but I recommend that if you are unsure you answer the question but select a *review* checkbox and go on to the next question. When you get to the end of the exam the software will present you with a list of all the questions you have marked for review. Bear in mind that you must complete all the questions within the time allowed for the exam, as at the end of the allocated time the screen will go blank and you will not be able to answer any further questions.

Once you think you have finished it is best to leave. Do not fill the time just going over the questions again, as it just leads to increased anxiety levels as you start to doubt some of the answers you were previously happy with. Remember though that if you are sitting in the morning session you will not be allowed to leave early.

Once you leave it is best to have something planned to occupy your mind. It is usual to chat with friends about the exam and no doubt this is what you have done before, but ask yourself if the post-exam dissections ever make you feel better about your performance. The answer is invariably no and the focus is inevitably on the more memorable questions which are usually the ones you all found very difficult.

Go shopping and treat yourself, spend some time with your family or friends. Do something positive that you enjoy and put the exam behind you. There will be plenty of time to reflect and dissect the paper at your leisure later.

Eve R (2003) *PUNs and DENs: Discovering Learning Needs in General Practice.* Radcliffe Publishing, London

Lewis S, Clarke M (2001) Forest plots: trying to see the wood and the trees. BMJ 322: 1479-80

Resources

Bandolier: www.jr2.ox.ac.uk/bandolier
British Hypertension Society: www.bhsoc.org
British Medical Journal (BMJ) www.bmj.com
British National Formulary (BNF): www.bnf.org
British Thoracic Society: www.brit-thoracic.org.uk
Clinical Evidence: www.clinicalevidence.com
Control of Substances Hazardous to Health: www.hse.gov.uk/coshh/index.htm
Data Protection Act 1998: www.opsi.gov.uk/ACTS/acts1998/19980029.htm
Driver and Vehicle Licensing Authority (DVLA): www.dvla.org.uk
European Computer Driving Licence: www.ecdl.nhs.uk
GMS contract: www.opsi.gov.uk/si/si2004/20040291.htm
GP Notebook: www.gpnotebook.co.uk
Lancet: www.thelancet.com
National Institute for Clinical Excellence (NICE): www.nice.org.uk
Pearson Vue: www.pearsonvue.com
Royal College of General Practitioners (RCGP): www.rcgp.org.uk
Scottish Intercollegiate Guidelines Network (SIGN): www.sign.ac.uk
UK Resuscitation Council: www.resus.org.uk

CHAPTER 4

The workplace based assessment

Although workplace based assessment (WPBA) is of course an important element of the nMRCGP, it is not actually a test as such and is by far the least challenging part of the overall assessment. However, you do need to complete it, there are some pitfalls, and some candidates will need a period of additional training due to its unsatisfactory completion. Another important point is that you can use some of the elements of WPBA to help you improve your performance in the other parts of nMRCGP, especially the clinical skills assessment.

The workplace based assessment is an online portfolio with entries mainly completed by the trainee but with input also from the clinical and educational supervisors. At the end the educational supervisor will conduct a final review which will essentially be a pass/fail decision. We will cover more detail on this later. The decision is both qualitative and quantitative, meaning that you can fail if your work is not to the required standard or if you simply have not completed all the required components of it.

There are several reasons why WPBA is required, the most important probably being that it assesses competency areas that cannot reliably be assessed in the other parts of the exam. There are important aspects to being a doctor that require more than just a snapshot assessment as can be delivered via the applied knowledge test and the clinical skills assessment, such as professional values and teamwork.

There are quite a few elements of the WPBA that are more concerned with formative assessment than the summative process of deciding whether you pass or fail. Formative assessment refers to an assessment that is used for the benefit of the learner, usually in the form of structured feedback, while summative assessment refers to an assessment that has a pass or fail decision attached to it. This handbook will attempt to focus mainly on those aspects which pose a potential threat to overall success in the exam, although some coverage will be given to the remainder.

It is somewhat unusual to combine formative and summative elements within the same assessment, the major concern raised being that if the learner knows his trainer is making a judgement as to his performance he will be less likely to own up to his weaknesses. The counter argument to this is that the distinction is somewhat artificial, as GP trainers have always completed a trainer's report which is essentially summative in nature.

It seems clear that the development and maintenance of an online portfolio is going to be a core feature in revalidation for GPs, so it is worth using the WPBA as an opportunity to develop the skills required for reflective learning. You should resist the temptation to record mere facts — for example listing all the articles you have read, tutorials attended etc. — and to instead focus on the ones that were meaningful to you and tease out what the important learning points were for you. You should also consider which ones might have stimulated learning that is generalisable to different scenarios.

4.1 The competency areas

The College has defined 12 competency areas for WPBA. They are listed below but a detailed discussion of each will not be provided as there is plenty of information about them on the College website:

- Communication and consultation skills
- Practising holistically
- Data gathering and interpretation
- Making a diagnosis/making decisions
- Clinical management
- Managing medical complexity
- Primary care administration and information management and technology
- Working with colleagues and in teams
- Community orientation
- Maintaining performance, learning and teaching
- Maintaining an ethical approach to practise
- Fitness to practise.

4.2 The educational supervisor

One significant change in this system of assessment has slipped through rather quietly — that is the introduction of an educational supervisor to provide continuity throughout the training in hospital posts. Previously a trainee who had four 6-month posts would have four consultants who would be both clinical and educational supervisors. Although arrangements are likely to differ throughout the UK it is likely that the vast majority of those in specialty training for general practice during their hospital posts will have a consultant as their clinical supervisor and a GP trainer as their educational supervisor. When the registrar gets to general practice the GP trainer will act as both clinical and educational supervisor. By the time you read this book it is likely that you will already be a long way through this process.

The consultant acting as clinical supervisor will retain responsibility for carrying out the various assessments detailed in this chapter, but the trainer acting as educational supervisor will be responsible for providing an overview, working with the trainee to develop a learning plan, make sure their portfolio develops appropriately, ensure that they engage with their clinical supervisor and that the various assessments take place. The educational supervisor will also be responsible for the supervisor's reports.

4.3 What the workplace based assessment is designed to assess

The WPBA aims to assess the issue of professional values. This encompasses all the attitude aspects of being a doctor:

- Caring and compassion
- Honesty
- Self-awareness and attitude to being a lifelong learner
- Motivation and ability to work within a complex team.

A good GP trainer will always have a good idea of how well his or her registrar is performing, and much of this impression is formed based on the informal observation of multiple sources of data: entries in records, informal comments by patients and staff, engaging in tutorials and of course by direct observation of the consultation, usually achieved by watching video recordings. The goal is for WPBA to make these assessments much more explicit and much more objective. This chapter will explore the various tools developed for this purpose, which are:

- Multi-source feedback (MSF)
- Patient satisfaction questionnaire (PSQ)
- Consultation observation tool (COT)
- Case based discussion (CbD)
- Direct observation of procedural skills (DOPS)
- Mini-clinical evaluation exercise (CEX)
- Clinical supervisor's report (CSR)

The evidence gathered for the WPBA, throughout training as well as through outcomes from the applied knowledge test and clinical skills assessment, is recorded in a web-based portfolio. The ePortfolio can be accessed by the trainee and the educational supervisor who will both be able to make entries in appropriate areas within it. Evidence from external assessments will also be recorded and the WBPA will not be able to be signed off until the applied knowledge test and clinical skills assessment have been passed.

4.3.1 Multi-source feedback (MSF)

Multi-source feedback enables the gathering of views about a registrar from several colleagues. The process is scheduled to take place twice in Specialty Training Year 1 (ST1) and twice again in Year 3 (ST3, which is the year in general practice).

During each multi-source feedback you will need to select five colleagues with whom you work and ask them to complete an online questionnaire about you. Your trainer will be responsible for ensuring that the sample of colleagues contribute to it, but he or she will not be aware of the raw responses.

The questionnaire consists only of two questions asking for an overall rating of the registrar's overall professional behaviour and clinical performance, along with space for both positive and negative free text comments.

Once complete the results will be sent to the trainer for debriefing. The results will be in the form of mean, median and range of scores for the rating scales and the anonymised free text feedback. You will discuss the results of the questionnaires with your trainer in a meeting and any reflections based on this will be recorded in the ePortfolio learning log.

As such you cannot actually fail multi-source feedback, but any serious concerns could result in a referral to more senior Deanery personnel. Serious concerns could arise either as a result of adverse scores and comments in the feedback or of a failure to respond positively to the discussion with the trainer. Both of these should be easy enough to avoid by reviewing the wording of the questionnaire forms (available to download from the College website) at an early stage in training and by thinking about how you should behave to elicit positive responses. It may be helpful to ask your trainer for informal feedback on a regular basis.

Similarly, the discussion with the trainer need not be a cause for concern; if there are any issues raised by the questionnaire your trainer will work with you to identify strategies to improve your performance and skills. Multi-source feedback were originally developed as a tool to help an individual improve rather than as a way of testing and you should not lose sight of this.

A little self-awareness is important when selecting the respondents. Throughout your training you should always try to gauge how others feel about you and respond to you, and it would be wise to apply some careful thought as to whom you invite to complete your feedback questionnaires.

4.3.2 Patient satisfaction questionnaire (PSQ)

For this exercise forms will be handed out on an agreed date to consecutive patients. The forms are anonymous and the patients do not give out any clinical information about themselves or their medical history. Patients will complete these questionnaires after the consultation and hand them back at reception. This continues daily until 40 patients have responded. The responses are then entered online by the Deanery staff. Even if these are entered independently there are still significant questions to be asked of this process as it is not blind. After completion of all the questionnaires there will be a similar feedback interview with the trainer as in during the multi-source feedback.

To generate serious concerns in the patient satisfaction questionnaire should surely require considerable effort! The feedback forms are downloadable from the College website and you will see that they are very focused on your patient-centredness, i.e. listening skills, appearing caring, explaining clearly and involving/empowering the patient. Although we all have an innate self-awareness of how good we are at these skills the way to make sure you score highly is to explicitly consider them when watching yourself on video and discuss your performance with your trainer. Sometimes these are skills that we use selectively — they are more difficult to use for example when you are stressed or very busy, therefore perhaps you should be selective about when you hand out your questionnaires and maybe a busy Monday morning is not the best time! You will of course be aware when they are being handed out and therefore be able to focus on being patient-centred and avoiding the kind of behaviour that is likely to result in patients scoring you less highly. Being polite and a good listener will go a long way, but will not be enough on its own.

4.3.3 The consultation observation tool (COT)
You are expected to have six consultation observation tool submitted to your ePortfolio for each of the final 6 months of your training, so by ST3 year you should have 12 completed. Consultations can be assessed by live observation but most are expected to be video recordings. Getting six done in 6 months does not sound terribly demanding but it is easy to let time slide and end up with frenetic activity trying to get them all done within a week or two, which will significantly impact on the amount of benefit you get from them.

The trainer will assess each consultation according to the consultation observation tool performance criteria. These criteria are very closely aligned to the old MRCGP video criteria which is good news as it means that even if you have never met them before your trainer probably knows them quite well. The criteria cover five different areas within the consultation:

- Discovering the reasons for the patient's attendance
- Defining the clinical problem
- Explaining the problem to the patient
- Addressing the patient's problem
- Making effective use of the consultation.

Your trainer will use these criteria to form an overall judgement on your consultation. The following grades will be used:

- Excellent
- Competent
- Needs further development
- Insufficient evidence.

The last of these grades is used where evidence for a specific criterion does not appear in the consultation in question and therefore does not necessarily indicate a sub-standard consultation, for example a consultation where there is no prescribing decision-making.

The trainer is expected to record feedback and recommendations for further development, and at the interview when the consultation is discussed you are expected to agree an action plan for improvement. The grading of your consultation observation tool is used to inform your trainer's overall decision for the final review; having a couple graded as 'needs further development' does not necessarily mean an automatic 'fail'.

There has been considerable discussion about the fact that your own trainer will be making this assessment, but working out a feasible methodology for external assessment has been fraught with problems and despite initial suggestions that at least one other assessor (another trainer or course organiser or programme director) is involved in rating a few of the cases there is currently no formal requirement for this and at present your trainer can complete all of them.

Again this is not a tool expected to 'fail' registrars; it is intended to give feedback and specific pointers towards improvement. The key will be in ensuring that the grades demonstrate improvement during the year from 'needs further development' towards 'excellent' nearer the end of the year.

However, a very important point is that although the consultation observation tool is not going to be perceived as a terribly high hurdle — the clinical skills assessment will probably be considered by most to be the most challenging part of the nMRCGP — it is very important that you gain all you can from the formative feedback you receive during the consultation observation tool process since this will prepare you for the clinical skills assessment. The marking criteria for the clinical skills assessment are quite different from the consultation observation tool but the same principles of patient centred consulting apply. For that reason we will explore the consultation observation tool criteria a little further, although there will be more discussion of consulting techniques in the clinical skills assessment chapter. The College website has a detailed guide to the performance criteria so the following section will be a relatively simple guide.

One important suggestion to make at the beginning is that there are pitfalls in using the 'consulting-by-numbers' approach of trying to attain the performance criteria individually without paying regard to the overall intention of what you are supposed to be achieving, namely that you end up with a dysfunctional, unnatural feeling consultation that appears to trainee, trainer and patient alike as being stilted and wooden. A good consultation can achieve the criteria while still having a natural flow. It may be helpful to think carefully about the five main headings as well as the individual criteria since they convey what the criteria are supposed to be achieving.

Make sure you use your trainer as a resource during your teaching sessions and indeed in the video feedback sessions using the consultation observation tool. Make sure you ask how your trainer would have done something if you do not think you did it well. Some trainers will be prepared to video record some of their own consultations and you might find these very useful (most trainers will not volunteer to do this but few will refuse if asked!). An alternative is to ask to sit in with your trainer and watch some of his consultations. All registrars sit in with their trainer during the very early part of their time in the practice, but you are in a position to be aware of so much more of what is going on in the consultation when you have more experience.

Remember that this is not just about surviving an assessment, it is about being a good doctor and it is easy to lose sight of the value of the video criteria and merely see them as boxes to tick. These subtle communication skills will stand you in good stead throughout the remainder of your hopefully long career in general practice.

The consultation models

Before discussing the video criteria in more depth it is worth reviewing consultation models. Dozens of books and hundreds of papers have been published on communication skills, and British general practice probably leads the way in this field. This chapter cannot possibly be a comprehensive guide to communication skills for general practice, but I will try to cover the most important aspects and try to incorporate elements from them in the discussion of the video criteria. The consultation models will also feature in the chapter on the clinical skills assessment.

I am not going to suggest you go away and read lots of other books either, but there are a couple of key texts you really must read and be aware of. You should hopefully be aware of them anyway, and they should be in the practice library of any self-respecting training practice.

Some of the earliest published work was written in the 1950s by Michael Balint. He worked with some London-based GPs and analysed what was going on in the consultation. He published his observations in his book titled *The Doctor, his Patient and the Illness,* first published in 1957 (re-printed in 2006). This work was important as it came at a time when general practice had fairly low status and people were just starting to consider the psychology of the doctor-patient relationship. I will not attempt to describe the book in any detail here and it is a fairly weighty tome that does not appeal to many GP registrars, but Balint wrote about the feelings doctors had when they consulted patients and how identifying the way a patient made a doctor feel could be quite important. He also encouraged doctors to meet together to discuss these feelings, what they meant and what they could do about them. He also wrote about the fact that a doctor himself could act in the same way a drug — with benefits, side effects and the potential for dependence!

In the 1970s Patrick Byrne and Barrie Long listened to 2,000 audiotaped conversations and identified six stages of the consultation (Byrne and Long, 1976):

Byrne + Long

1. • Establishing a relationship
2. • Identifying the reason the patient came
3. • Conducting a verbal and/or physical examination
4. • Doctor and/or patient consider the condition
5. • Doctor and patient agree on further treatment or investigation
6. • Doctor closes the consultation.

Importantly, they identified that problems in phases two and four of the list above were most likely to lead to 'dysfunctional consultations'. They also described the terms 'doctor-centred' and 'patient-centred'.

In 1979 Nigel Stott and Robert Havard Davis described the primary care consultation as consisting of four parts (Stott and Davis, 1979):

- Management of presenting problems
- Modification of help-seeking behaviour
- Management of continuing problems
- Opportunistic health promotion.

Although nowadays generally considered very doctor-centred, this model does promote holistic care and is the only model to include an element of demand management within it.

The Consultation — An Approach to Teaching and Learning (1984) was written by Pendleton, Schofield, Tate and Havelock. The important concept of 'ideas, concerns and expectation' first appeared in their book. Their book also describes the use of a video recorder to analyse and teach consulting skills and described seven tasks:

- To define the reasons for attendance, including the nature and history of the problem, their aetiology, the patient's ideas, concerns and expectations, the effects of the problems
- To consider other problems: continuing problems at risk factors
- To choose with the patient an appropriate action for each problem
- To achieve a shared understanding of the problems with the patient
- To involve the patient in the management and encourage him to accept appropriate responsibility
- To use time and resources appropriately
- To establish or maintain a relationship with the patient which helps to achieve the other tasks.

Although written by four authors this model is generally referred to as Pendleton's model. In addition to introducing ideas, concerns and expectations the patient-centred concepts of achieving shared understanding and involving the patient in the management also appear.

The Inner Consultation by Roger Neighbour et al (2004) describes a five stage process:

- Connecting
- Summarising
- Handing over
- Safety netting
- Housekeeping.

Although it is the five stages people remember best there are lots of other important observations in Roger's book, making it important reading for all GP registrars.

Finally, *The Doctor's Communication Handbook* by Peter Tate (2006) summarises most of what is in the other books, along with plenty of helpful material. It is very easy to read and is a very practical and pragmatic guide to consulting, with Peter's personality and wealth of experience as a GP trainer coming across clearly. I strongly recommend you read this book even if you do not read any of the others as you should be able to read through it in a couple of evenings and I am sure you will find it is time well spent.

It is worth noting that Pendleton, Schofield, Tate, Havelock and Neighbour have all been heavily involved in the MRCGP exam and its development over the years. You can interpret this in different ways but whichever way you look at it the College's exam has always had strong links with the development of 'the consultation'.

We will now get back to the consultation observation tool performance criteria.

Discovering the reasons for the patient's attendance
A detailed guide to the consultation observation tool performance criteria is available on the College website. You will see that the section on discovering the reasons for the patient's attendance contains four criteria:

- PC1: The doctor is seen to encourage the patient's contribution at appropriate points in the consultation
- PC2: The doctor is seen to respond to signals (cues) that lead to a deeper understanding of the problem
- PC3: The doctor uses appropriate psychological and social information to place the complaint(s) in context
- PC4: The doctor explores the patient's health understanding.

Although these criteria are of course each important individually do not to lose sight of the overall aim of this section, which is all about finding out why the patient came to the surgery and what their ideas, concerns and expectations are — think back to the Pendleton consultation model described above.

We have known for many years that there is a strong correlation between accurately identifying and addressing the problem the patient has come about and achieving a positive outcome to the consultation, be that measured by patient satisfaction or otherwise. It requires active listening skills and the ability to be able to encourage the patient adequately without interrupting. Some of the information may be conveyed non-verbally, so you need to be on the lookout for facial expressions, body language, pauses and have the ability to apply your own non-verbal skills to explore the patient's agenda. This includes putting the patient's problem into a social and psychological context, which is beyond asking what they do for a living or who lives at home with them. You need to demonstrate genuine interest and really try to find out what is going on inside the patient's head, what makes them tick and how the problem affects the patient's life in their normal daily activities.

When a patient knocks on your consulting room door do you remain seated, stand until they sit or go over to the door and shake their hand? You probably have an innate style that influences this, and there is not a right or wrong approach. It is likely though that while some patients will welcome a more formal approach this may lead to a more formal doctor-patient relationship. There are times when you may want that, but perhaps not always.

The opening part of any consultation is very important as there are so many different ways of doing it. If you have read Roger Neighbour's book *The Inner Consultation* you will know that what a patient says when they first walk into the consulting room and how they deliver it can convey more information than is given in the words alone. In the clinical skills assessment the role-players are carefully briefed to deliver their opening statement in a highly standardised way. All role-players playing an individual case will therefore use exactly the same form of words.

Roger Neighbour describes the curtain raiser — a spontaneous and unintended remark made by a patient as they enter the room — and argues that it often tells you a little more about what is going on in the patient's head than the statement they have been rehearsing while in the waiting room. While it is of course entirely possible for the case writers to script this sort of thing into the role-player briefing, in the vast majority of cases the patient will have a simple opening statement telling you why they have come. For example: *'I've been having a pain in my stomach doctor'*, or *'I've been worried about these headaches I've been getting'*.

Have you thought about the effect your greeting has on a patient? Have you tried experimenting with different approaches? There are lots of ways of starting a consultation and each is likely to have a different effect on the patient, even when it is a simulation. A traditional medical approach is to directly ask the patient why they have come, with a statement such as: *'Hello Mrs. Jones, what's been the problem?'*, or *'What can I do for you today?'* or *'How can I help?'*, which can in real consultations save some time as it avoids preamble about the weather. A more open and encouraging approach is to open the consultation with a less direct question or statement, such as: '*How are you today?*', or '*Hello, I'm Dr. Jones*', or '*I don't believe we've met before*'. You can even actually say nothing but smile and gesture for the patient to sit down. This allows the patient to say what they have rehearsed without you distracting them and tends to make them feel a little less hurried. What is important is that you experiment with the different styles to observe the different responses they elicit and to establish a technique and form of words that you personally feel comfortable with. If you can open the consultation confidently and smoothly both you and the patient will feel better about it and will therefore be more likely to volunteer the information you need more easily.

As medical students and during junior hospital jobs as young doctors we tend to develop bad habits that are hard to break later; we learn our history taking as a series of formulaic questions, initially relying on a fairly rigid structure of pretty much entirely closed questions. As GPs we need to become comfortable with a less formal structure, with a more compact focused history and with much more use of open questions. You will need to concentrate on trying to only ask open questions during the early part of the consultation at least and not interrupting the patient. A commonly quoted study found that doctors interrupted patients after 23 seconds on average (Marvel et al, 1999). As doctors we are worried that if we just let the patient talk they will go on for ever, but this is not usually the case. Other studies have demonstrated that if uninterrupted, patients conclude their initial 'monologue' within 30 seconds on average within primary care (Rabinowitz et al, 2004). Try it yourself and see; you will generally find they run out of steam quite quickly and some patients will actually get uncomfortable doing all the talking and will want you to contribute. Learning the skills to encourage and facilitate the patient's initial contribution is important and using your video feedback sessions with your trainer is an important way of doing this. Using your videos it is quite easy to observe how long you let patients speak before interrupting them and how good you are at using open questions.

It can be disheartening as a registrar to keep asking patients what they think might be wrong only to get very non-committal answers at best or '*You're the doctor*' at worst! You need to ask yourself why it is that patients are not prepared to own up to what they are worried about and think about how you can address that. Generally speaking, patients are acutely aware that you know far more medicine than they do and are therefore afraid of appearing silly if their ideas are off the mark. They may also be afraid you will think they are hypochondriacal and/or neurotic. Some patients feel it might be presumptuous for them to tell the doctor what they think the problem is, particularly the less well educated. Therefore when you ask what they think the problem might be they shrug and say they do not know, then when you tell them what you think it is they say '*Yes, I thought it might be that!*'. Denial can be another reason for patients withholding their thoughts from you; although they have considered a diagnosis they are not actually prepared to articulate it, to you or even to themselves.

The trick here is to get the patient to trust you, and there is no simple form of words that can be offered as suggestions; it is important that you develop your own ways of achieving this based on your own personality and style. Very often you can second guess what the patient is worried about, for example (and these are of course generalisations), patients with headaches are often worried about brain tumours and strokes, patients with chest pain are worried about heart attacks and blood clots, etc. You can utilise this by speculating out loud, for instance: '*I wondered if you had any worries that it might be something serious like a brain tumour*', or '*People with these sort of symptoms are often worried it might be their heart...*'. Experiment and find phrases that you feel comfortable with, trying not to make it sound formulaic as if it feels uncomfortable to you it probably will to the patient too and you will get nowhere. The timing of your enquiry is also important; it is no good asking the patient what he thinks the problem might be early on in the consultation and it is better to leave it till a little later when you have had a little more chance to establish rapport. Another trick is to slip the question in when the patient is distracted by something else, for example during the examination.

Remember that one of the commonest things patients say about a doctor they like is that he or she really listens to you. Being a popular doctor is not the be all and end all, but it is very rewarding when patients like you and come back to see you for the right reasons. The doctor who is the good listener is far more likely to find out the real reasons why patients come to see them and discover their innermost thoughts and worries.

To satisfy PC3 requires more than just seeking out psychological or social information — the criterion specifically refers to using this information to put the complaint in context. For example, rather than simply enquiring what work the patient does you should find out exactly what that entails and how their medical problem impinges on it. Often patients say what their work is without it meaning much to you, for example a patient might say he is a 'diesel fitter' but asking what this actually entails might reveal that his work involves maintaining commercial vehicles with lots of heavy lifting.

Exploring the patient's health understanding has already been pretty much covered already but it is worth reminding you that the criterion requires that you actually explore rather than just find out what the patient's own ideas are.

Defining the clinical problem
This section comprises of three performance criteria:

- PC4: The doctor obtains sufficient information to include or exclude likely relevant significant conditions
- PC5: The physical/mental examination chosen is likely to prove or disprove hypotheses that could reasonably have been formed or designed to address a patient's concern
- PC6: The doctor appears to make a clinically appropriate working diagnosis.

The section is thus about attempting to make an accurate diagnosis. To do this you need to make appropriate hypotheses about differential diagnoses and ask the right questions to include or exclude likely conditions, followed by an appropriate examination. You must demonstrate the requisite medical knowledge to direct your questions and your examination. Note the use of the words 'likely' and 'significant'. Experience with the MRCGP video examination has led to concerns that some registrars concentrate on the communication aspects of the consultation to the detriment of the practical clinical skills and decision-making. It is important that you know the right questions to ask to home in on the problem and that you do so efficiently.

Having been exhorted to use open questions and not to interrupt the patient, one of the problems registrars run into is that they are not sure when to stop using silence, listening and using open questions and when to take charge of the consultation and get on with the more closed medical questions. The consultation then ends up a bit disorganised and loses focus.

Sometimes it can be helpful to flag up specifically to the patient that you are going to move into a different phase of the consultation. Once you are happy that you have gathered enough information regarding the patient's concerns it can be helpful to reflect back to them your interpretation of the reason they came. For example you might say something like: '*Just to be sure I have understood correctly, you have come about these headaches you have been having in the evenings, and you were worried they might be due to something serious?*'. Do not get into the habit of repeatedly summarising though as this leads to a disjointed and dysfunctional consultation.

Once you have ascertained that you have understood correctly you can indicate that you are going to take charge a bit more, asking something like: '*Would you mind if I ask you some rather more medical questions now about your symptoms?*'.

You must make sensible choices in deciding what examination to carry out. The second part clearly acknowledges that sometimes we perform an examination more because the patient is likely to expect it than because we perceive that it will yield useful information. For example a patient with what you think are tension headaches will perceive your examination to be incomplete if it does not include a blood pressure check, even if the patient's blood pressure has been recorded recently.

When you come to examine the patient get into the habit of asking permission and explaining what you want to do and why in plain language, for example: '*Would it be OK if I popped you onto the couch so I can feel your stomach?*'. It is also helpful if you give the patient a commentary of what you are looking for as you examine.

It is particularly important that you flag up any aspects of the examination that might be uncomfortable or which might be misinterpreted. Even a simple examination like fundoscopy can appear odd to a patient if they do not know what to expect or why you are doing it. Remember also to ask the patient if they would like a chaperone, especially if you are examining women or children.

Use some common sense in deciding if an examination is OK to be seen on camera. Clearly an intimate examination such as a breast examination must be off camera, either out of shot or by covering the lens, but not every exposure of flesh requires this. If you cover the lens for simple examinations, for example examining a child's chest or looking into their ears, your trainer might be worried about what you are trying to hide! There is the additional factor that switching off or covering the camera reminds both the patient and yourself of the camera's presence, possibly increasing self-consciousness on both sides. If you are not sure about your examination technique then ask your trainer for some help with it rather than trying to conceal your weaknesses. Just make sure you conduct a clinically appropriate examination.

Remember that you are training to be a GP, not a specialist, so choose a focused examination that is likely to help you in your decision-making and/or reassure the patient that you have examined them satisfactorily. This is not your medical student finals so you are not generally expected to conduct a full cardiovascular examination or a full neurological examination (unless it is really appropriate). Do however use the correct techniques for the examination you do carry out, and do not do silly things such as listening to a child's chest through a duffle coat!

The final criteria in this section is about the actual working diagnosis you make. Remember that the assessor (and indeed sometimes the patient) cannot always make a judgement about the appropriateness of your diagnosis unless you make it clear what that is, so it is good to get into the habit of making sure you always explicitly verbalise this to the patient. You can also of course record your working diagnosis in the consultation log.

Explaining the problem to the patient
There are two performance criteria in this section:

- PC8: The doctor explains the problem or diagnosis in appropriate language
- PC9: The doctor specifically seeks to confirm the patient's understanding of the diagnosis.

The first point to make is that of course you must make an effort to explain the problem to the patient. When explaining your diagnosis the commonest problem is the use of medical jargon, and you will almost always find you are using more than you think you are. The only way you are likely to pick this up is by watching yourself on video and looking for it specifically. One of the problems again is that patients do not want to appear stupid. So when you say, for example: '*I can see some conjunctival erythema*', they are likely to nod sagely and pretend they understand exactly what you are talking about when they may in fact not have a clue. Saying: '*The white of your eye looks a bit red*' is more user-friendly and conveys just the same information.

While it is important to use plain English to explain a diagnosis or problem to a patient, many patients do also like to know the actual medical term for their diagnosis, so it is useful to also give this. If you write it on a piece of paper for the patient this allows them the opportunity to look it up for themselves on the Internet later, or discuss it with friends/relatives.

At this point you will be rewarded with even more brownie points if you refer back to the patient's health ideas in your explanation. Apart from impressing your trainer it makes the patient feel like you have listened to them and care about their concerns. This is not terribly difficult, you just need to get into the habit of doing it and it is well worthwhile as you will find you achieve more in your consultations. An example might be to say: '*I know you were worried you might have a chest infection and need some antibiotics, but I'm reassured by the fact that you don't have a temperature and your lungs sounded nice and clear when I listened to them*'.

You will need to make sure the patient has understood your explanation. This is difficult to do well at first until you find effective ways of doing it. Certainly just simply asking if the patient has understood will not suffice as they will generally collude with you to make you happy, and asking them outright to explain the problem back to you really does not work well as it makes the vast majority of patients feel very uncomfortable — if you have ever watched this done on video you do not need to look too carefully to see the expression on the patient's face and their body language, they often visibly squirm in their seat. Think through the problem here; patients do not like admitting they have not understood your explanation as they do not want to appear stupid themselves and also they do not want to offend you by suggesting that your explanation was incomprehensible!

Experiment with different techniques and avoid formulaic phrases, for example: '*What are you going to tell your wife when you get home?*'. Although this can work if done well, it often results in the patient looking at you as if you have just landed from Mars.

It can help to suggest that what you explained was a bit complicated and difficult to understand and offer to clarify any bits they did not quite get, or even to suggest that sometimes you find it difficult to explain the problem clearly and that you would be happy to go over it again. This will help the patient feel it is not their fault they did not understand and will make them more inclined to ask for clarification.

Addressing the patient's problem
This section contains two performance criteria:

- PC10: The management plan (including any prescription) is appropriate for the working diagnosis, reflecting a good understanding of modern accepted medical practice
- PC11: the patient is given the opportunity to be involved in significant management decisions.

Make sure your management plan is medically appropriate and that you can justify any investigations, prescriptions or referral, by reference to evidence and guidelines if possible. As a GP in training there is an understandable emphasis on patient safety. Do not make the mistake of assuming that the consultation observation tool is purely about communication skills — your medical knowledge is important.

You are expected to involve the patient in decision-making and this is something you need to start practicing early on as it is something you are unlikely to have done in your hospital posts. Again do not just think of it as something to do to keep your trainer happy as it is a genuinely useful tool to be able to use in the consultation; it means your patient is more likely to leave the consulting room happy and more likely to comply with whatever management plan you have agreed. It needs to be done selectively, and there will be times when it is appropriate to be fairly doctor-centred and directive, for example when you suspect the patient has a serious condition, but it is usually still possible to involve them in the decision-making to some extent. It is important also not to start offering the patient options that are inappropriate, for example antibiotics for a simple uncomplicated cold.

There are lots of occasions when the way forward is not clear-cut and where more than one approach can be justified. Many would argue that this applies to most problems in general practice. Patients appreciate having the situation explained to them and being involved in the decision-making process. It can also help make your life easier – two heads are often better than one and sharing the responsibility can reduce your own anxiety and stress levels.

The threshold at which you either wait and see or treat/refer is rarely black and white and the patient's opinion can usefully be taken into consideration. We all have different personality traits — some patients really do not like investigations or taking tablets while others would like to intervene early. If you are not certain what to do it can be helpful explaining this to the patient and exploring their personal preferences.

Involving the patient in the management decision does not necessarily mean doing what they want. There are many other factors to take into account, such as our responsibility to other patients and to use resources sensibly. It does not also mean abdicating your responsibility to the patient — if there is a difficult decision it is your responsibility to help the patient to understand the issues and to be able to contribute to the decision but if the patient wants to leave it to you as a health professional that is their right. It is unfair to ask a patient to make a decision when they do not feel they have sufficient background knowledge.

Making effective use of the consultation
There are just two performance criteria in this final section:

- PC12: Makes effective use of resources
- PC13: The doctors specifies the conditions and interval for follow-up or review.

There are many facets to making effective use of resources, one of the most valuable being your own time as a doctor: practice being efficient; recognising when you have enough information to move the consultation forward; asking focused questions rather than wasting time; not asking lots of questions which do not actually contribute to the decision-making process. One key difference between experienced doctors and trainees is that experienced doctors tend to be more decisive, recognising when they have gathered enough information, whereas trainees often tend to start repeating questions and going round in circles. This then confuses the patient and undermines your own confidence when you realise you are doing it! If you think you have gathered most of the relevant information but still are not absolutely sure what the problem is or how to move forwards what you need to do is stop and think rather than gathering more information which often tends to lead to confusion or the exploration of 'blind alleys'. Do you need to allow more time to see if the problem either resolves or evolves? Do you need to arrange some investigations or refer? Is a trial of some treatment appropriate?

Other obvious resources are NHS resources — prescribing and the referral to others either within the extended primary care team or in secondary care. Working as a GP within the NHS does bring with it responsibility for managing resources effectively, and although you may feel uncomfortable with the gate-keeping role it is an integral part of your job as a GP. It must of course be balanced with your role as the patient 's advocate and it can be very difficult balancing an individual patient's needs with the wider needs of the NHS and society.

Beauchamp and Childress described a framework of medical ethics in 1978 which is widely referred to and contains the following four elements:

- Autonomy
- Beneficence
- Non-maleficence
- Justice.

Beneficence and non-maleficence are best thought of as 'doing good' and 'doing no harm', and in the context of making effective use of resources the balance to be struck is between the competing demands of patient autonomy and justice. The patient's autonomy is their right to self-determination and their right to have the best available treatment for themselves, but of course with the limited resources available within the NHS this can impinge on the resources available for other patients — distributive justice

It is surprising how many consultations close without the patient being given a clear indication as to when they should come back. If you feel you need to see the patient again then say so clearly (next week, in a month, in six months, etc.). Sometimes you need to give conditional instructions, offering earlier review if there is a deterioration or if a drug causes side-effects. There are specific instances where giving patients instructions on when to return are particularly important; for example when seeing an ill child it is important to give the parents very specific indicators to looks for which might indicate a need for early review. When prescribing a drug which sometimes is not tolerated very well, for example an antidepressant, it is sensible to arrange to review early so the drug can be changed if need be.

An important skill not specifically addressed by the performance criteria is that of closing a consultation. Sometimes there is a natural conclusion to a consultation, particularly when handing over a prescription or giving advice on when to come back, but sometimes you need to politely indicate that the consultation is drawing to a close. In practice this is often done by simply repeating a summary of the advice already given or the follow-up instructions, but another techniques is to take the opportunity to check that you have dealt with the patient's problem satisfactorily and that the patient has understood your explanation and instructions. A sentence such as: *'I think that just about covers things for today Mrs. S, unless you have any questions?'*, combines a clear indication that you feel it is time to end the consultation with an opportunity to clarify anything not understood.

4.3.4 Case based discussion (CbD)

This tool is designed for use during both the hospital and practice based components of training. The idea is that the trainee documents a case which is then used as the basis for an interview with the trainer/supervisor. The purpose is to explore professional judgement in situations of complexity and uncertainty, applying medical knowledge, ethical and legal frameworks and prioritising appropriately. Justification of decision-making will be sought.

To make things easy the trainee chooses a selection of cases for discussion, although the assessor will decide which ones to discuss. There are to be six discussions during each training year for ST1 and ST2, with 12 in your general practice year. The case paperwork has to be made available to the assessor beforehand so he can plan questions he wishes to ask. There are no specific criteria as to which cases the trainer should choose, but trainers are likely to choose cases that look like they have more scope for discussion, so it is likely to be the more complex cases or ones where the trainer felt perhaps that you could have handled the case differently.

The case based discussion paperwork is all downloadable from the College website, including the guidance to trainers on formulating structured questions. Again this is not something you can actually 'fail' although the interviews will contribute towards the final workplace based assessmen; remember that this is largely about formative assessment so the discussions are a learning experience with some assessment thrown in. Good case-based discussions can be challenging and really make you think.

First of all you need to select your cases. It is probably best not to go for completely straightforward cases as there will be little to discuss and you will get nothing out of the process, not to mention the fact that you will get little credit as they will not demonstrate much to the assessor. On the other hand you do not want to select cases you think you made a mess of, unless you are confident you have analysed what went wrong and are confident you can suggest better ways of managing the problem. Very complex cases may not be such a good idea as they can take a lot more than the recommended 20 minutes to discuss, the result then being that you risk having a fairly superficial discussion skating over lots of issues without discussing them in any depth.

When you write up the cases it should be easy enough to work out what issues are likely to come up. Work systematically through the case starting with the history:

- Did you ask all the right questions? Is there anything else you would have liked to ask in retrospect?
- What examination did you choose and why? Did it contribute to making a diagnosis?
- What investigations did you choose and why? What else might you have done and why did not you choose that? Make sure you consider the evidence base behind your decisions and justification
- How did you come to your working diagnosis, what else did you consider and what influenced your decision-making process?
- How did you decide on your next management steps? What other options did you have, and can you discuss the implications of each?
- Try to think of what challenges your trainer could pose to your decisions and how you might justify the decisions you made.
- If you felt you lacked some knowledge that might have helped you how have you addressed this since?
- When considering implications think broadly: implications for whom? Consider the implications for the patient, yourself, the practice team, the NHS generally
- Was there any ethical aspect to the case? If so can you tease this out and discuss your decisions in the context of an ethical framework?
- How did you elicit the patient's views? How did you incorporate them into the management plan?
- How did you feel after the consultation: did you find it stressful? If so why and how did you deal with that? How do you think the patient felt leaving the consulting room?

Your experience during the discussion will depend to some extent on your trainer — there is quite a bit of skill required from his point of view and some trainers challenge their registrar more than others. Unless he or she really is much cleverer than you there is no reason for anything to come up in the discussion that you have not already thought of, after all you supply the cases and get a chance to prepare them.

It is important that you do not consider the case based discussion just an academic exercise. The skills being tested are really important to you if you are to be a good GP. It is good to get into the mindset of asking yourself the questions above on a regular basis until you are able to incorporate them into your live decision-making processes while you are with a patient. If you can do this it will stand you in good stead when you come to sit the clinical skills assessment.

4.3.5 Direct observation of procedural skills (DOPS)

Direct observation of procedural skills is an assessment of specific clinical skills that you will need to be a GP. They are intended to be carried out throughout the three years of your training, so you might already have completed some or all of them before starting your year in general practice. These are fairly minor assessments and it is not expected that you fail any of them — if one is unsatisfactory it should simply be repeated. They are listed below. There are eight mandatory procedures that all trainees must be observed in:

- Application of simple dressing
- Breast examination
- Cervical cytology
- Female genital examination
- Prostate examination
- Male genital examination
- Rectal examination
- Testing for blood glucose.

There are also eleven optional procedures:

- Aspiration of effusion
- Cauterisation
- Cryotherapy
- Curettage/shave excision
- Excision of skin lesions
- Incision and drainage of abscess
- Joint and peri-articular injections
- Hormone replacement implants
- Proctoscopy
- Suturing of skin wound
- Taking skin surface specimens for mycology.

The two lists above should be reviewed on the College website as there was considerable change from year one of nMRCGP to year two, and it is likely they will continue to evolve.

4.3.6 Mini-clinical evaluation exercise (CEX)

Six Mini-clinical evaluation exercises per year are to be carried out during hospital posts as an alternative to consultation observation tool, which often is not possible in the hospital setting. However as this is still very much in the development phase it could be possible that COTs might eventually be done in hospital too. Since this book is aimed at those in ST3 we will not go into any detail.

A mini-clinical evaluation examination is an observed interaction with a patient to assess your clinical skills, attitudes and behaviours. Following the debrief the assessor will provide feedback and during the discussion areas for improvement will be identified and recorded. Each encounter will need to cover a different clinical area.

4.3.7 Clinical supervisor's report (CSR)

Although entitled clinical supervisor's report it seems that these will actually be completed by your educational supervisor — remember in some areas this will be your GP trainer, and in others a different GP trainer to the one you will be with for you year in general practice.

Every six months your educational supervisor will need to conduct a review of your progress to date, collating the evidence gathered from the various assessments and complete a report. You can download a copy of the paperwork for this from the College website.

During the review you will complete a self-assessment in addition to the trainer performing an assessment of your progress in the 12 competency areas set out at the beginning of this chapter.

The assessment part of the report has three main areas:

* Knowledge-base relevant to the placement
* Practical skills relevant to the placement
* Professional competencies — which breaks this down into the 12 competency areas.

At the end of training the educational supervisor conducts a final review following which he makes a recommendation to the Deanery regarding your competence. There is no self-assessment at this final review and in the final review the educational supervisor must 'grade' each of the 12 competency areas, the grades available being 'insufficient evidence', 'needs further development', 'competent', or 'excellent'. The form can be viewed at the College website and it is essentially a tick box section.

If the trainer feels you are not competent in any area an expert Deanery panel will look at the evidence and adjudicate.

4.4 The ePortfolio

The concept of using an educational portfolio in medicine is not new, indeed they have been in use in postgraduate general practice for well over a decade.

The term portfolio in this context derives from the world of art and design, where a student would over the course of his training collect pieces of his work in a portfolio. This would then be assessed to gain qualifications and would be used as a showcase of work to demonstrate the artist's skills.

Early general practice portfolios arose from doctors recording experiences they had encountered in their workplace that identified a learning need. A key element of the process was the reflection required to tease out the learning needs from the event and deduce an appropriate method of meeting the needs identified.

As the Internet developed, so have electronic portfolios. One of the benefits of these is that access control can be implemented to allow various different personnel to access and sometimes contribute to the portfolio, based on secure account authentication. Thus in the case of workplace based assessment the registrar and the trainer can contribute directly to the portfolio while external bodies such as the College and Deaneries can contribute outcomes from external assessments. The final outcome can provide proof of completion to both College and Deanery to provide final certification as a GP.

It is recommended that you also read the relevant pages on the College website and the documentation provided within the ePortfolio section and review them periodically as the workplace based assessment is constantly evolving and no book can hope to be up-to-date.

4.5 How to ensure success

You can see from all these sections that the assessment throughout the workplace based assessment is very closely linked to the teaching, much of it occurring in teaching-type sessions. Feedback therefore will be continuous and you should know at an early stage if you are falling short of the mark in any areas and should be able to work with your trainer to ensure any weaknesses receive special attention to rectify the situation. You will not get to the end of your training to find your trainer unexpectedly finds himself unable to recommend your competence!

To get into general practice specialty training you must have demonstrated sufficient aptitude that you are capable of comfortably passing all the elements of described in this chapter. The major challenge is to make sure this fairly onerous schedule of assessments gets fitted into your placements. Clearly this will be your responsibility although your trainer will share this with you and will endeavour to keep things on track, working in partnership with you. You are going to need the co-operation of the consultants and specialist registrars you work with during your hospital placements, and although your trainer will be there to help with this you need to engage with them throughout your training. Make sure you try your best to 'get on' with all the people you work with and maintain regular communication with your trainer.

The workplace based assessment is not a terribly challenging hurdle from the point of view of degree of academic difficulty, it is more a question of motivation, diligence and application. For most GP registrars the major perceived hurdle will be the clinical skills assessment and do not lose sight of the fact that there is huge overlap between the competencies you need to demonstrate during workplace based assessment and those required for the clinical skills assessment.

Beauchamp TL, Childress JF (2001) *Principles of Biomedical Ethics.* 5th ed. Oxford University Press, Oxford

Marvel MK, Epstein RM, Flowers K, Beckman HB (1999) Soliciting the patient's agenda: have we improved? *JAMA* **281**(3): 283–287

Rabinowitz I, Luzzatti R, Tamir A, Reis S (2004) *BMJ* **328**(7438): 501–502

The clinical skills assessment

The Clinical Skills Assessment (CSA) appeared in 2007 as an entirely new assessment. It shares many features with the old MRCGP simulated surgery component, but there are differences. As has been mentioned previously it is expected that registrars will perceive this to be the most challenging hurdle within the nMRCGP, and it is entirely possible that perception proves to be reality.

As its name suggests, the clinical skills assessment is a test of clinical skills, and they cannot be taught in a book like this. What this book can do however is give you as full an understanding of the assessment as possible: what it is designed to assess, how it actually works, how the cases are designed, and how you will be assessed, in addition to guidance on how to prepare for and maximise your performance in the examination.

The range of problems you could face in the clinical skills assessment is almost infinite, just like the range of cases you might face in a surgery in general practice. However the broader nature of the problems and the competencies required to deal with them is much smaller, and what we can do in this chapter is identify and discuss the many themes arising. This may appear confusing but will hopefully become clearer later on in the chapter!

5.1 What it is designed to test

The stated purpose of the clinical skills assessment is: '...*an assessment of a doctor's ability to integrate and apply appropriate clinical, professional, communication and practical skills in general practice*' (Royal College of General Practitioners). What this means is that it will test your competence in these skills by actually making you demonstrate them in a standardised environment. It will test your ability to actually apply knowledge in a clinical scenario.

The clinical skills assessment provides a variety of standardised cases so that the degree of challenge is controlled by the examiners rather than by yourself; there is an objective, criterion-referenced marking schedule and the grades are decided by a series of independent, highly trained, experienced examiners. Criterion referencing means that your performance is compared against a predetermined level of competence rather than against other candidates — it does not matter how well or how badly others do, and if you perform well enough you pass.

The clinical skills assessment is thus about far more than just communication skills. Once you have gathered information about why the patient came to the surgery, you must use this along with your medical knowledge to make appropriate clinical decisions and formulate an appropriate management plan. The information gathering may include a physical examination of the patient. The consultation must be conducted in a patient-centred way, seeking out and acknowledging the patient's own ideas about the problem and potential solutions and involving them in the decision-making. Your professional values may come under scrutiny, for instance your ability to recognise ethical dilemmas and resolve them satisfactorily.

As stated on the College website the clinical skills assessment aims to test you in the following areas:

- Primary care management: recognition and management of common medical conditions in primary care
- Problem-solving skills: gathering and using data for clinical judgement, choice of examination, investigations and their interpretation
- Demonstration of a structured and flexible approach to decision making
- Comprehensive approach: demonstration of proficiency in the management of co-morbidity and risk
- Person-centred care: communication with patients and the use of recognised consultation techniques to promote a shared approach to managing problems
- Attitude aspects: practising ethically with respect for equality and diversity, with accepted professional codes of conduct
- Clinical practical skills: demonstrating proficiency in performing physical examinations and using diagnostic/therapeutic instruments.

5.2 When to sit the clinical skills assessment

The first thing to discuss is when you are actually going to sit the assessment. The main sittings are from January through into February and in May. In 2007 and 2008 there were additional sittings in the Autumn (September or October). Subject to demand further additional sittings can be slotted in if required. There is a balance to be struck here: sit it too early and your chances of failing are much higher, but if you leave it until the last sitting before completing training there is a risk you will fail and be unable to start work as a GP.

The following advice applies assuming your training includes just one year in general practice and your ST3 year starts in August — if you started in February or some other time, or if you are training part-time, you will need to adjust accordingly. If your final year is in general practice I would strongly advise that you do not even consider the October sitting since your chances of passing are slim unless you are some sort of prodigy!

It is tempting to sit in January or February so that should you fail you still have the opportunity of re-taking the exam in the May sitting. I think however that becoming proficient in the skills we have detailed in this chapter by February and getting it all into ten minute consultations only halfway through the year is a bit of a tall order and that your chances of passing are significantly higher in the May sitting. The failure rate of candidates sitting towards the end of their training is expected to be very low. Of course if your scheme includes 18 months in general practice as is expected to become the norm then sitting in the January/February is quite a reasonable option as you will then have spent a full year in general practice.

Should you fail on your first attempt the cost to re-sit the exam will be the same whether you take the exam in January/February or in May. Your chances of passing are however significantly higher later on, reducing your risk of having to pay the examination fee a second time. Should you fail in the May sitting however there is the added complication that you cannot start work as a GP until you re-take the exam and pass, and you would not be able do that until September or October. You then have the option of seeking funding from your Deanery for additional training (which is the ideal) or simply treading water until September/October. Circumstances in Deaneries will vary, but the Deanery has already invested a lot of time and money into your training, and they have already given you a form of endorsement via the selection process you underwent to get onto the training scheme in the first place, and they are unlikely to abandon you at this stage. However you should discuss this with both your trainer and your course organiser/programme director.

5.3 The format of the exam

The examination is in the form of a simulated surgery. You will sit in a consulting room and see a series of 13 simulated patients. You will have a maximum of 10 minutes to consult each patient, with a short break of about two minutes between each consultation and a break halfway through.

You will be provided with a brief patient record which may detail any previous relevant or significant medical history, current medication, perhaps brief records of recent consultations, investigation results or hospital letters. The record will be as brief as possible to avoid burdening you with unnecessary information and is unlikely to fill a single side of A4. You will be able to read the record in the gap between consultations.

At the start of a consultation the patient will knock and enter the room and the consultation will begin exactly as it would in your usual surgery. If you have not finished by the time the buzzer sounds after 10 minutes is up the patient will get up, say goodbye and leave.

5.3.1 How the cases are designed

There are several ways simulated patient scenarios can be devised. The first thing to say is that the scenarios are all devised by experienced case writers, all of whom are experienced examiners and GPs. Some have had previous experience in writing cases for the simulated surgery in the old exam, but all have had training in writing cases. Cases are generally written in pairs firstly as it can be a bit isolating sitting on your own writing cases, but mainly because two heads really do work much better than one in all aspects of writing the case — coming up with ideas, spotting possible problems and pitfalls and in refining the actual wording.

One obvious way of writing cases is by drawing from experience; typically a writer might experience an encounter with a patient in which something happened that made it stand out as a suitable case. Generally speaking this would be a consultation that featured a specific challenge. The writer then needs to tease out the specific issues raised by the case and trim out any extraneous features that complicate it.

The next step is to identify what this case would be testing by reference to the curriculum statements and link it with one or more specific intended learning outcomes, or ILOs. Alternatively, the writer must identify (or be given) a curriculum statement to write a case for, and then choose specific intended learning outcomes. The case writer then needs to consider possible clinical scenarios that would test in that specific area. This technique is useful when the management team identify that a particular area of the curriculum is short of cases.

The majority of cases are derived by the former method, i.e. based on an examiner's experience of a case since this is much easier to do than 'working backwards' from a specific curriculum statement and it tends to naturally produce a more realistic and valid case.

There are three separate elements to the case writing. The first of these is defining what the case is designed to test and what the case writer expects a registrar to have to do to pass the case. The second part is the role player briefing, which defines clearly the age and sex of the role player, the presenting complaint and quite detailed guidance on how to dress, how to behave and how to release information. The final part is of course the examiner's marking schedule which will specify which domains the case tests and what you are expected to do in each to pass.

Case writers face several challenges. While you clearly do not need to appreciate all the intricacies of writing the cases, understanding these challenges can help you prepare for the exam. The most important is probably to make sure that the case feels real, important to both you as the doctor consulting the patient but also to the role-player. For you as the doctor it is important that you feel that the patient sitting in front of you is real, and that the problem they present feels just like the sort of thing you face in your day-to-day surgeries. You must be able to get into consultation mode and forget that it is an examination. For the role-player it is important that they can identify with the case and put themselves completely into role and play it naturally without having to think through it too much as they go along.

It is important that the scenario is sufficiently tightly focused, making sure it tests what it is set out to and that it does not present too many opportunities to wander off down blind alleys that are not relevant to the marking schedule. The case writers also must ensure that the case can be completed in the allocated time, or at least cover most of it within the 10 minutes you are allowed. This means avoiding too much complexity while retaining an appropriate level of challenge — a case that is too straightforward and presents too low a challenge does not discriminate sufficiently between good candidates and weaker ones.

The marking schedule must be meticulous. It is very important that it leads the examiner observing the case to reward the correct consulting behaviour and conversely that it does not reward inappropriate behaviour. It can be difficult to make sure that the candidate cannot get sufficient marks just through a mechanistic history taking and examination.

The cases all have to be piloted before they can be used in a live examination. It is impossible to be certain a case will work as planned; some cases fizzle out quickly and the level of challenge needs to be raised, others prove to be too complex for candidates to handle in 10 minutes. Often the role-player briefing needs tweaking to ensure the description of symptoms enables the good candidates to make a correct diagnosis or to modify the advice to the role-player on the level of 'cueing' to offer. Sometimes symptoms need to be trimmed to avoid candidates following false leads. Similarly the marking schedule will invariably need some adjustments to reflect the reality of how the consultation actually plays out in reality. The aim is to present you with a patient who presents in as realistic a way as possible and gives you the opportunity to demonstrate your consulting and clinical skills.

5.3.2 What you are likely to meet

Theoretically you could come across any medical problem during your surgery in the clinical skills assessment. However, there are some constraints that can help you narrow down the range of what to expect.

You will not encounter any of the very simple, straightforward and often trivial problems patients often present us with in our day-to-day surgeries in general practice. Although this would add realism, it would add little in the way of helping the examiners discriminate, and at the end of the day that is what an exam is for, to discriminate between candidates from poor through to excellent. Discrimination is generally perceived to be a bad thing in current society, but in this context of course it is not a bad thing as long as the discrimination is both reliable and valid.

There are huge limitations on what physical examinations the examiners can expect you to perform in the consultations. One limitation is that it is unreasonable to expect the role-players to undergo intimate examinations, or anything that might be considered uncomfortable or the least bit invasive. This even excludes some apparently simple procedures such as checking blood pressure, for which the General Medical Council have issued specific guidance as to how many times a day it is considered reasonable for this to be done on a patient. Also, because this is a licensing examination it is important that all candidates experience a standardised challenge, so any physical signs must be as near as possible to identical for all candidates. This means that using real patients with physical signs as happens in other exams is a problem so physical signs will need to be either simulated by the role-player (for example simulating pain or tenderness, a restricted range of movement of a joint, etc.) or using the sort of models or artificial body parts you may have encountered previously in Objective Structured Clinical Examinations (OSCE). However, the clinical skills assessment is designed to test your integrated clinical skills, unlike an OSCE where for example a station might involve a single element of an examination, for example checking the blood pressure.

Despite a desire on the part of the College (and Postgraduate Medical Education and Training, PMETB) to assess your clinical examination skills, in reality this accounts for only a small part of the assessment. The majority of what you will be assessed on will be your communication skills, your ability to integrate your findings and medical knowledge, to formulate a diagnosis and then generate a suitable management plan.

The examiners would also like to present you with urgent medical problems, but again there are significant limitations as to what can reasonably be simulated. For example, they cannot realistically present you with a patient who is short of breath, but it is certainly possible to present you with a patient with acute pain who may require urgent management. You should not assume that because it is a simulation a patient could not possibly require an urgent intervention, such as hospital admission.

There are several different aspects to a consultation and this chapter will deal with these in separate sections. Of course in a consultation lots of these merge together and are not performed sequentially, but for the purpose of teasing out everything that goes on and how you can become better it is helpful to identify them separately. Here are the basic components of a consultation:

- History taking
- Examination (physical or mental)
- Making a diagnosis
- Explaining the diagnosis
- Formulating a management plan.

5.3.3 The patients
All the role-players receive training before playing a role in the examination. Currently the role-players are chosen from a single agency that also provides

role-players for other medical exams, and most of the role-players are already highly experienced. In addition to 'generic' training for their work with the clinical skills assessment, every role-player will have specific training in the individual role to be played which will involve watching video footage of the role being played in its piloting or in a previous live exam. There is a also a lengthy session before the exam every morning involving all the examiners and role-players involved in each case during which the role-players rehearse and fine tune their performances with guidance from the examiners.

A lot of time is spent ensuring that the role-player not only presents the case accurately to you but also that it is done in a highly standardised way so that it is played in an identical way to every candidate. This means not only using the same form of words but includes the emotional level it is presented at — some roles require the patient's mood to be low, anxious, upset, angry, and minor differences in how this is played can have a major effect on the experience that you as a candidate have. Role-players have to be carefully rehearsed in how they are expected to react to what you as a doctor might do or say in the consultation.

All of this detail is provided to reassure you that you can go into the assessment confident that you will be presented with a series of realistic patients and that they will consult with you in exactly the same way as with the candidate in the next room, the day before and the next week, etc. Their job is to present you with a standardised challenge, to play the case accurately without either unduly helping or hindering you. You can just get on with the job of being as good a doctor as you can during your 10 minutes with them without worrying about them tripping you up or misleading you.

Age

You will meet a variety of patients of both sexes and with a wide range of ages. At the time of writing there are no cases involving the use of children as role-players since there are practical difficulties in using children (related to length of working hours and missing school), so any cases involving children will involve a parent coming to see you about the child in the child's absence. There is however no reason why children might not appear in the future. All the patients you meet will be professional role-players, many but not all of whom may be professional actors.

The role-player's age is generally carefully matched to the suggested age of the patient they will be playing. Sometimes this may just be an age range, for example 40 to 50, but for some roles the age of the patient may be quite critical.

To help address the difficulty of using very young and very elderly role-players the patient's and role-player's age may not always match exactly. For instance a role-player in their late 60s may play an 80 year old, or an older teenager may play a younger role. In these cases a lot of effort will be put into ensuring a performance that makes the age of the patient appear credible using dress, make up, etc.

Social class

As well as age and sex mix, the case writers try to provide a balance of social class, from highly educated and articulate patients through to working class or unemployed and relatively poorly educated patients. Remember however that generally speaking trained actors are fairly well educated and are invariably articulate, and while they are good actors and can compensate for this to some extent where required it is fair to say that the majority of patients you will meet in your clinical skills assessment surgery will be articulate and middle class.

Ethnicity

There will be a mixture in terms of ethnicity, in some cases the patient will happen to be Asian or Afro-Caribbean but their ethnicity will be coincidental to the role. In other cases however the patient's ethnicity or cultural background may be a key feature of the case requiring you to specifically address any issues raised by this.

5.4 The greeting

When a patient knocks on your consulting room door do you remain seated, stand until they sit, or go over to the door and shake their hand? You probably have an innate style that influences this, and there is not a right or wrong approach. It is likely though that while some patients will welcome a more formal approach this may lead to a more formal doctor patient relationship. There are times when you may want that, but perhaps not always.

The opening part of any consultation is very important — there are so many different ways of doing it. If you have read Roger Neighbour's book *The Inner Consultation* (referred to in Chapter 4) you will know that what a patient says when they first walk into the consulting room and how they deliver it can convey more information than is given in the words alone. In the clinical skills assessment the role-players are carefully briefed to deliver their opening statement in a highly standardised way. All role-players playing an individual case will therefore use exactly the same form of words.

Roger Neighbour describes the curtain raiser — a spontaneous and unintended remark made by a patient as they enter the room — and argues that it often tells you a little more about what is going on in the patient's head than the statement they have been rehearsing while in the waiting room. While it is of course entirely possible for the case writers to script this sort of thing into the role-player briefing, in the vast majority of cases the patient will have a simple opening statement telling you why they have come. For example: '*I've been having a pain in my stomach doctor'*, or *'I've been worried about these headaches I've been getting'*.

In chapter 4 we described a number of ways of greeting the patient at the start of a consultation and discussed the varying effects they might have on the subsequent consultation. The clinical skills assessment is however a little different. First the role-player has a carefully rehearsed opening statement that will not be dependent on how you greet them and start the consultation. Second these are patients you have not met before and you are in a formal exam setting so it is best that you greet them relatively formally by introducing yourself and confirming that they are indeed the patient you expect them to be. It can often appear a little more formal if you go to the door to greet the patient and it perhaps gets the consultation off to a smoother start if you remain seated and just allow the patient to come in and sit down unless there is a specific reason, such as a disabled patient who may need some assistance. The consequence of a clumsy and uncomfortable start is that the patient will feel less comfortable and you are likely to have to work much harder to gain the patient's trust.

Roger Neighbour describes five checkpoints in the consultation. The first is 'connecting', meaning that you should establish rapport with the patient. Rapport means establishing a relationship with the patient, empathising with them and establishing mutual trust and respect. It is often difficult to pitch your initial behaviour with a patient since they all tend to have slightly different expectations and values. For some the doctor-patient relationship is a formal one, particularly for elderly patients. Others prefer a much more informal and personal relationship where using the patient's first name would be more appropriate that their surname. One constant is that you need to appear friendly and while some of this is about smiling as you greet it is also hugely dependent on your body language. This can be difficult in an exam situation where you are feeling anxious and tense so it will require some positive effort to try to appear relaxed and welcoming.

The role-players will react to you exactly as a patient would, so making them feel welcome and putting them at ease is important. There is a balance to be struck however, and it is important you do not overdo it and appear over-enthusiastic or excessively cheerful! It is also possible to appear smarmy or patronising and you need to watch yourself on video to judge if you are getting it right.

5.5 Taking the history

Once the consultation is under way you can get down to the nitty-gritty of finding out why the patient came. As a medical student you will have learned a very structured approach to medical history taking which involves asking lots of closed questions and is very doctor-centred. As a GP you need to move on from this — that is not to say that you can forget all about what you originally learned, but you certainly will not get through much of a routine history and examination in the 10 minutes you are allowed. More importantly, however, you are also likely to miss out on lots of important information. Therefore as well as developing a more focused technique you must become more patient-centred to ensure you discover all the psycho-social elements to the problem as well as uncovering any hidden agendas.

A lot of the information can be gained for free, without you putting any effort at all in, and it is important that you maximise this. When patients see a doctor they already have lots of information available to give you and it is important to let them do just that! The first technique is to simply not interrupt the patient. This sounds easy but it is something many doctors find very difficult to actually put into practice. It is easy to understand why this is — we are worried that if we just let them talk they will go on forever, but we just cannot resist butting in and elaborating the details of the first important thing they say. As already described in Chapter 4, doctors interrupt their patient after about 23 seconds on average and patients generally talk for no longer than 90 seconds before appearing to seek doctor input, suggesting that we overestimate the amount of time patients will talk if left to it. It is quite difficult to change this behaviour, so do not wait until you turn up to the assessment before trying it. You need to practice this in your normal surgeries, preferably while video recording so you can observe how long you can actually go before you intervene and so that you can try to appreciate the value of the information volunteered. It is also important to learn to do this appropriately — if you just sit there saying nothing most patients will feel uncomfortable and will probably clam up. So you need to develop what are known as active listening skills and develop a feel for when the patient does want you to respond or take a little more active control of the consultation.

Active listening

Active listening means that while listening you are taking some positive steps to encourage the patient to talk. This is generally in terms of non-verbal communication, although often encouragement is vocalised as '*mmmmm's*', '*uhuh's*', etc. If you look disinterested or frankly bored the patient will predictably not take this as encouragement. Posture is important; when interested in what someone has to say we generally lean forward, but you need to appear relaxed at the same time or it can appear a little intimidating. An open posture usually means with hands relaxed in your lap or on the desk rather than with arms folded.

Eye contact is important; it is no good gazing off over the patient's shoulder, staring at a computer screen or written records or fiddling with your pen. Make it clear the patient has your undivided attention. We also use more subtle facial expressions to make it clear we are listening carefully; sometimes cocking the head to one side, but perhaps more importantly responding appropriately by nodding, frowning, or raising eyebrows. Again it is important that all this is done in a natural way, and if overdone it can be very destructive! Watch yourself on video, ask for feedback from your trainer or other colleagues, and watch others consult if you get the chance so you can observe for yourself what you think works and what does not.

Asking further questions

Where you do feel the need to ask further questions you should firstly try to store them in your head to ask when the patient has finished speaking and always try to ask open questions rather than closed since this allows the patient more freedom to express themselves. The first principle is to try to avoid asking questions that lead to a '*yes*' or '*no*' answer. Ensure that your question encourages the patient to give more detail, for example: '*Can you tell me a bit more about the pain?*', rather than: '*Was it a sharp pain?*'. Use the techniques described in the previous paragraph to encourage the patient and make sure you give them time to answer.

Using silence

Using silence is an important consulting technique — it can feel uncomfortable and it is sometimes difficult to resist the urge to break the silence either by rephrasing your question or by asking a different question. Remember that if a patient does not understand your question or cannot think of an answer they will usually say so.

Silence in a patient indicates usually that they are thinking of an answer, and are taking some time either because it is something they feel uncomfortable talking about or because they cannot find the right words to express it. Often the silence will be accompanied by loss of eye contact, the patient often lowering their head. You should keep looking at them so you can resume eye contact when they look up. If you do eventually feel compelled to break the silence there are ways of doing this that can give the patient further encouragement, either verbally by acknowledging their difficulty or non-verbally, by touch for example.

Just as in real-life, patients in the clinical skills assessment may not always present in a straightforward way — they may present you with multiple symptoms or their initial presenting complaint may not actually be the main problem (we will specifically discuss hidden agendas later in this chapter). Patients presenting with a list of symptoms can be challenging to deal with and you need to have strategies for dealing with this.

One approach is to take each item in the list at a time and while this may seem appealing there are drawbacks. First, you are unlikely to have enough time to work your way through any kind of list in the 10 minutes you have with the clinical skills assessment patient. Second, this approach often misses the point — a list of symptoms that appear unconnected to a patient may actually be different manifestations of the same underlying problem (for example a patient presenting with tiredness, low mood, poor concentration and irritability). A useful strategy can be to gather all the symptoms together to see if there is any obvious pattern.

It might be worth asking the patient if they think they might be connected.

If the symptoms do not appear connected and it genuinely appears the patient is presenting with multiple different problems then you need to prioritise. Patients do not generally mean to make life difficult for us, and often are not consciously aware that when they book an appointment with us it is for a finite length of time. They also sometimes underestimate the difficulty of some of the problems they throw at us. It is OK to explain to a patient that you have limited time with them and that you might need to arrange another appointment to deal with some of the problems. This needs to be handled sensitively, avoiding making the patient feel short-changed or as if you are fobbing them off. Patients will understand that trying to deal with lots of problems in a single 10 minute appointment will mean you cannot really do justice to any of them and will lead to a superficial handling.

There is a risk that a patient may be made to feel stupid if your response comes across in the wrong way; you may not mean to sound like you are saying '*You can't possibly expect me to deal with all that lot in one go!*', but it can seem like that if you do not get it right. It can sometimes be helpful to 'take the blame' yourself, making it sound like a weakness of your own rather than of the patient.

5.5.1 Prioritising the problems

You must involve the patient in the prioritisation, even though it may be obvious to you which problem should be dealt with first. Saying something such as: '*I think I'll struggle to deal with all those problems properly in one go -- was there one in particular that you'd like us to address first?*' might be one approach. Or: '*Shall we have a go at dealing with the most important problem and see how we are for time after that?*'.

When it comes to spotting hidden agendas there are lots of strategies you can use. Those who argue that consulting is an art rather than a science would perhaps have you believe that the good doctor has a kind of 'sixth sense' for this sort of thing and just gets a feeling that there is something more there. Whilst it is difficult to disprove this, it is probably more likely that the good doctor is just more expert at spotting the more subtle clues, generally non-verbal ones. The good doctor is probably also that little bit more suspicious that there could always be something going on in the background and actively seeks clues. It does seem that these skills appear elusive to novice consulters, so do not worry if when you start your year in general practice you do not feel as if you are 'tuning in' to much of the background agendas. Although there is no substitute for experience it is fair to say that experience alone will not be enough and that you certainly can learn the skills required. We will come back to hidden agendas later.

5.5.2 Patient-centred consulting

If you recall back to chapter two patient-centred consulting appears prominently in the curriculum. Being patient-centred is not about doing what the patient wants, it is about really tuning in to the patient, finding out about why they came, what exactly it is about their problem that is worrying them and what sort of solutions they thought you might be able to offer.

The term 'ideas, concerns and expectations', often shortened to ICE, refers to the fact that patients almost always have their own ideas about what might be wrong with them, the seriousness of their symptoms and their implications and they almost always come with expectations as to what you might be able to do. Patients pretty much always have their own ideas about what is behind their symptoms, but GP registrars often find it difficult discovering what those ideas and health beliefs are. That is because finding this out actually is quite difficult!

You may ask patients what they think might be causing their symptoms and more often than not they will simply tell you they have no idea. Then later when you tell them what you think the problem is they will say: '*Yes, I did wonder if it might be that*'. Why do patients do this? This is more common in patients from the lower socio-economic groups — you often find that the more educated patients are all too willing to tell you exactly what they think the diagnosis is, and possibly even what management they expect too, sometimes all of it in the opening 30 seconds of the consultation. For many patients an encounter with a doctor is not exactly threatening, but they certainly do not feel on an equal footing with you. They are acutely aware that you are a highly trained professional who of course knows far more about medical problems than they do, and as a consequence they are very self-conscious about their ideas and worry about divulging them to you: they may be worried they might be just plain wrong and therefore that you will think they are stupid, they may be concerned that despite their worries you will find that there is nothing seriously wrong and you will therefore consider them neurotic, or they might have a stereotyped view of what a doctor patient relationship should be like and be concerned that you will consider them presumptive for considering a diagnosis.

You will need to learn a few tricks to get patients to spill the beans. The first point is not to ask too bluntly. Asking simply: '*What do you think it is?*' will almost invariably result in a shrug and a denial. You need to be a little more subtle and ask a little more indirectly. More open questions can be helpful. Asking something like: '*What have you made of all of this?*', or '*Do you have any theories about what might be causing it?*' sometimes does the trick since it implies their ideas are more tentative. Another strategy is to ask what their family have made of it, that way it is the family who potentially look stupid or neurotic rather than the patient themselves. Timing can be important: asking very early on in the consultation is less likely to be effective and asking during the main history-taking phase of the consultation makes it seem a more important question whereas if you can slip it in as an aside a little later, for instance when they are getting on the examination couch or during the examination, it can be disarming and may be more likely to result in a frank answer. Again your tone of voice, facial expression and body language are important and you need the patient to believe that you really do expect them to have some ideas of their own and that you will value and respect those. A plea for help can sometimes be fruitful, for instance: '*It would be really helpful to know what you think about it*'.

Often it is not difficult to second-guess what the patient's self-diagnosis might be, or they might even have hinted at it, in which case it is easy to offer something such as: '*Did you wonder if it might be ...?*'. It is often worth a stab in the dark even if you have no idea what they are thinking since it might still provoke them into volunteering some information. A statement such as: '*People very often have a good idea about what's wrong with them*' sometimes helps.

Once you have identified what the patient's self-diagnosis is it is important that you treat it with the respect it deserves, even if you think they are wrong. You should acknowledge what they have said and you really must explicitly include it in your discussion of the diagnosis. It is often helpful not to challenge it straight away as this can make it appear that you are either dismissing it without due consideration or are jumping to conclusions. Far better to wait until you have finished your information gathering and deal with it then, at which point you can congratulate the patient on having correctly identified the problem or tactfully explain why you do not think their diagnosis is correct. Saying something like "*I know earlier you said you were worried you might have a chest infection, well, I can see why you thought that, but ...*' is a way of suggesting that although they were wrong their suggestion was quite reasonable.

5.5.3 Identifying concerns

Identifying concerns is very similar but is subtly different. Early on in his *Doctor's Communication Handbook*, Peter Tate points out that patients invariably think their problem is more serious than you do, and this is always worth remembering. Again, asking patients directly about their concerns is not always helpful. Sometimes you can use cues, for example: '*You seem quite worried about it*'. Asking something such as: '*Do you have any particular worries?*' implies that you assume they do have worries about their symptoms but invites them to tell you about the most serious concerns they have.

The 'guessing what is in the patient's head' strategy can again be helpful. For example: '*Were you worried the headache might be due to a brain tumour?*'. Another approach is to depersonalise the problem, so you might say: '*Lots of patients with headaches worry that they might have a brain tumour. Did you?*'.

5.5.4 Pin-pointing the problem

Having hammered home the importance of patient-centred consulting, using open questions and exploring the patient's ideas, concerns and expectations, it is important that you do not overlook the plain old medical history taking. It is really important that you do ask the right questions about a patient's problem to make an appropriate medical diagnosis. A common pitfall in the simulated surgery has been for candidates to concentrate on the communication skills but fail to make a correct clinical diagnosis. One of the key skills you need to learn is when to 'shift mode' slightly in a consultation. In most consultations there does come a time to move on from the open questions and move into a more doctor-centred phase where you do ask closed questions to test your diagnostic hypotheses and exclude some of your differentials. It can be helpful to 'signpost' this shift to the patient (and even to the examiner!) by saying something such as: *'OK, I think I've got quite a bit of information to go on. Would you mind if I just asked you a series of questions to help narrow things down a bit?'*.

Occasionally a patient might take advantage of the opportunity to talk freely and carry on talking for what seems forever. Although most have some insight and at some stage will stop, this is not always the case. In these cases you will need to intervene to take control of the consultation. There is not a set time for this and it should be dependent on what the patient is telling you — once you feel the information they are giving you is not taking you forwards you will need to consider intervening. This might be because they are going round in circles telling you the same thing repeatedly, or describing repeated occurrences of the same symptoms or going off on tangents without focusing on what they actually came about. Although the 'patients' you will meet in the clinical skills assessment are generally very well trained and are not likely to do this spontaneously, do not overlook the possibility that this sort of behaviour might be written into the case to specifically test your skills in coping with it! There are different ways of dealing with this depending on the circumstances, and initially it can be best to just remain silent, withdrawing the earlier encouragement. If that fails it is probably generally better to deal with it explicitly rather than simply interrupting, for example by using a statement like the one at the end of the previous paragraph. Referring back to something they said earlier and asking for clarification can get things back on track while still valuing their contribution. You might need to acknowledge something else they have brought up and explicitly 'park' it and ask if it is alright to come back to that later once you have dealt with the main problem.

5.5.5 Summarising
Roger Neighbour's second checkpoint is 'summarising', which is a way of checking that you have correctly grasped why the patient came. The principle is that you summarise back to the patient what you think you have got out of them. Again you can signpost this to make it explicit what you are doing. For example say: *'Do you mind if I just check that I've understood correctly?'*.

The actual summary should be kept simple. For example say: *'So the main reason you've come is about the headaches, and you were a bit worried they might be migraine?'*. The benefit of this is that it can actually save you lots of time; it is surprising how often we think we have understood why a patient has come but get it wrong, resulting in a dysfunctional consultation where the patient leaves without you actually having addressed their problem.

The problem with identifying summarising as a useful technique is that it can lead to overuse! Avoid the temptation to summarise multiple times during a consultation unless you are genuinely confused and need to recap — apart from wasting valuable time patients can find it quite irritating when you keep repeating back what they have said.

5.6 Examining the patient

Once you have completed your history-taking the next stage of information gathering is generally to examine the patient. As has already been pointed out, the options in terms of presenting you with abnormal physical signs are somewhat limited. However, the examiners can still expect you to conduct a wide variety of clinical examinations.

An issue candidates seem to struggle with is uncertainty about whether they will be expected to actually examine the patient, examine a model as in an objective structured clinical examination or simply be presented with clinical findings either on a card or verbally from the examiner. It is generally best to behave as you would in a normal consultation and to proceed with whatever examination you think is appropriate at the time you would normally conduct it. You should simply ask the patient if they do not mind you examining them and take your lead from them. It is best not to look to the examiner for guidance — if the examiner has information to give you they will offer it when they feel appropriate, which may well be after they have watched you examine the patient.

Here are some key points to remember:

- Choice of examination
- Consent
- Technique.

Taking these in turn, the actual physical examination you choose to conduct is really important. This is an examination about general practice, so whatever you choose to do must be appropriate for a general practice consultation. It must be relevant to the patient's problem, and it must be likely to provide further information to help you make a diagnosis.

There is an important balance to be struck between being 'thorough' and focusing your examination to what is important and what can reasonably be fitted into a 10 minute consultation. You really do need to use your time efficiently and effectively, while at the same time satisfying the examiner that your examination is sufficient to assist you with your differential diagnosis. The important skill here is in knowing what actually will help you in your decision-making.

For example if a patient presents with a headache you might feel that to be thorough you should conduct a full neurological examination. You know however that you cannot possibly fit that into a normal general practice consultation, but do not worry because the examiner knows that too and will be assessing you as a general practitioner, not as a neurologist. The examiner also knows that depending on the actual history much of it is likely to be completely fruitless and a waste of your time. So perhaps you might focus down to checking the patient's blood pressure along with a few key cranial nerves, certainly including examining the fundi.

Occasionally an examination is conducted more to reassure the patient than because you think it might actually give you meaningful information. This would generally be to acknowledge a patient's presumed or elicited health beliefs. For example we know that a common health belief is that nose bleeds are a manifestation of high blood pressure, and therefore any patient presenting with a nose bleed is likely to expect to have their blood pressure checked. In this circumstance it is entirely reasonable to conduct an examination that may well not contribute particularly to your decision making. It is sometimes reasonable to sensitively address the health belief, for instance by explaining that high blood pressure does not generally cause nose bleeds but that you will check the blood pressure anyway to reassure them. You could argue that thus you are potentially reinforcing the health belief, but if you do not do it there is a risk of the patient leaving worried!

Think clearly about why you want to conduct a particular examination — practice doing this in your everyday surgeries, and after you have examined the patient reflect on what if anything it contributed. By the time you examine a patient you will generally have some hypotheses about the diagnosis, or a list of differentials. Your examination should be chosen to not only confirm or refute these hypotheses but also to exclude any possible serious conditions. If the examiner would prefer you did not subject the patient to a particular examination then either the patient or the examiner will advise you of this and it may even be pre-empted by information within the patient record on your desk (for example a recent blood pressure reading). However, if you choose to waste your time either performing an examination that is not likely to help you, or spend too long on an examination, the examiner is not there to help you out and is likely to let you carry on. If it is relevant you may be presented with information either to pre-empt you examining the patient of after the examination, giving you some physical signs either verbally or on a card. It is best to behave exactly as you would in a 'real' consultation — if you would like to examine the patient speak to the patient about it and do not ask the examiner or look to the examiner for cues.

For patients with psychological problems you would not generally conduct a physical examination but would instead conduct a mental state examination. Again this should be focused and appropriate to the patient's presenting problem.

5.6.1 Consent

If you do wish to examine the patient it is important to gain permission first. For the patient to be able to give informed consent they must have an understanding of what you intend to do, so you must start by explaining that you would like to examine them and explain what that examination will entail in terms of which part of their body and what form the examination may take.

Do not forget that what might be entirely routine to you may be completely alien to a patient. Try to put yourself in the patient's position and imagine what their fears of an examination might be (typically that it will either be embarrassing or that you will hurt them). It is important that you are honest — if an examination will cause an element of pain or discomfort do not tell the patient that it is not going to hurt. You are not likely to be allowed to conduct any intimate examinations within the clinical skills assessment so embarrassment is not likely to be a factor. You can safely assume that the examiner can act as a chaperone and you will not be marked down for not offering one.

Make sure that you are actually asking the patient if it is OK to examine rather than simply telling them. For example say: '*Would you mind if I had a listen to your chest?*', or '*Is to OK if I pop you on the examination couch and feel your stomach?*'.

You need to avoid the use of jargon and practice using plain English. This includes anatomical descriptions of where you plan to examine as well as any procedures or instruments you plan to use.

If your patient is a child this introduces a couple of other issues. First, you are dealing with at least two patients, both the child and any parents with them, so you need to make sure both understand what you would like to do and both are happy for you to go ahead. Second, children are likely to have a much lower level of understanding and less experience of medical examinations and any explanation must take account of this. Finally, children tend to be more afraid of doctors and are generally naturally more apprehensive so will need more reassurance that you will not cause them discomfort.

5.6.2 Technique

Once you have gained permission you need to go ahead with your examination. While this should be an examination appropriate for a general practice consultation, this does not mean it can be haphazard! You must have a clear idea of what you are examining and perform the examination in a systematic manner. Remember the general principles you were probably first taught when you were a medical student, and at all times treat the patient with courtesy and respect. Remember that the role-player will be playing this part over 20 times in a day and it is important that they are not hurt or damaged in any way. This may sound obvious but handling the patient in a rough manner is a sure-fire way of alienating them and giving a bad impression to the watching examiner.

The fluency with which you conduct the examination is important. You should be confident and relaxed as it helps both patient and examiner if you look like you know what you are doing rather than hesitating after each stage as you think through what you are going to do next.

The first part of the examination is to make sure you gain adequate exposure of the part you want to examine. For example, for a chest examination you really do need to ask the patient to remove their shirt or top, ditto for a shoulder examination. You will also want to be able to compare with the other side, particularly for a musculoskeletal complaint. There will generally be a predefined limit for this and if the patient says they would rather not remove an item of clothing you should not push this (they will have agreed with the examiner beforehand how much clothing is to be removed). Alternatively the examiner may direct you to examine the patient without removing a specific garment.

Next you should attempt to gain as much information as possible without touching. You should inspect quickly for anything obvious but remember that you are not likely to see any rashes, skin lesions, swellings or deformities in the clinical skill assessment. Although the role-players will not have obvious visible abnormalities, they will be very well rehearsed in demonstrating pain on movement, so they may have a limp or appear in some pain while removing clothing. Similarly they will reproduce a limited range of movement or pain on movement very reliably. If the patient's complaint includes pain ask them to point out the exact location for you. If the complaint is musculoskeletal you should elicit an active range of movements — this should be systematic and include all planes of movement. Remember flexion, extension, adduction, abduction and both internal and external rotation. When examining a limb you must always compare it with the other side. You must constantly monitor whether any of the movements are causing the patient pain by asking them to let you know and by watching their face as well as the part you are examining.

You do not need to give the examiner a commentary as you examine, but patients appreciate you explaining what you are looking for and why, and remember that commenting to the patient on any obvious abnormality ensures the examiner also knows you have spotted it!

Before actually laying your hands on the patient you should check if there is anywhere that is sore so you can avoid causing pain. Being considerate and gentle is paramount; ask the patient to let you know if anything you are doing is painful. You should palpate gently to identify any tender areas and check for any masses or swellings. In the case of joints you need to check the range of passive movements and look for any joint effusion. Depending on the area you are examining there may be specific manoeuvres to perform. There is a list of specific examination techniques you should revise later in this chapter. Again remember to always monitor the patient's face for signs of pain or discomfort.

Percussion and auscultation must be performed as appropriate, but you are unlikely to find any physical signs. It is important however to conduct them in a proficient manner: be systematic, practice your technique so it does not look like you have never done it before. This might sound patronising but you probably are not used to examining patients while being observed and assessed by a senior colleague, and most of us are aware that in our day-to-day practice we slip into bad habits and cut corners. Make sure you listen in the right places and that you look as if you would actually identify any physical signs.

As soon as you have finished examining let the patient know they can dress again as it is embarrassing sitting talking to someone when you are half undressed and even more embarrassing if the buzzer goes and the patient needs to leave the room undressed! Even if you have explained what you are doing as you go along, it is a good idea to summarise your findings to the patient at the end of the examination. Again you need to avoid using medical jargon and offer to explain anything the patient does not understand. We will cover explaining in a little more detail in the next section.

5.7 Diagnosis

In this section we will cover everything that comes after taking a history and examining the patient — this includes making a diagnosis, explaining to the patient, formulating and negotiating a management plan, prescribing and referral.

5.7.1 Making a diagnosis
It is worth taking a little time to consider how we actually make diagnoses as doctors. Early on in our careers we tended to take a comprehensive history and then examine the patient thoroughly before coming to any conclusions. That is not how experienced doctors do it though, especially in general practice where time is at a premium. What experienced GPs do is start considering hypotheses the moment the patient comes through the consulting room door. By the time the patient has finished telling their story a GP will generally already have a pretty good idea what is going on, and if they do not already have a tentative diagnosis they will have narrowed their list of differentials down significantly. Their choice of examination will be informed by this and they will focus very much on looking for physical signs that help them confirm their putative diagnosis, differentiate between different diagnoses and exclude any more serious conditions that they consider to be on the horizon.

There also tends to be a difference between the way GPs as generalists make diagnoses compared to their specialist colleagues. As generalists we consider problems in a broad context, integrating the psychological and social aspects with the physical medical ones. While we do still narrow down as we home in on a diagnosis (this is done on the basis of probability rather than exclusion), generalists tend to be more tolerant of uncertainty. Generalists tend to make their diagnoses by building up an overall impression based on many different factors, each of which contributes a small part of the information being processed.

An example would be a patient presenting with chest pain: a generalist would assess the problem based on the nature of the pain, the patient's age/sex and other contributory risk factors such as whether the patient was a smoker, obese, had an adverse family history, etc. While it might be possible to completely exclude the pain being cardiac, a generalist who considered it to be a very low probability would be comfortable exploring other options without needing to instigate other investigations such as an ECG or blood tests. A specialist would be more likely to want to collect evidence that provided more concrete proof that it was not cardiac.

The differences in approach have important implications for use of the doctor's time and other expensive resources as well as for the patient in terms of exposure to unpleasant investigations and generation of higher levels of anxiety.

Of course GPs do still often need to arrange further investigations and this applies to the clinical skills assessment as it does in normal consultations. Think carefully about whether your investigations are a critical step that prevent you from discussing a management plan and make sure you do not use them as a way of avoiding a difficult decision or discussion. Make sure you explain clearly to the patient what investigations you want to request and why, and restrict yourself to investigations that will be helpful — do not make the mistake of thinking '*I've filled in the form now so I may as well tick a few more boxes*'. Make sure you explain a clear plan for discussing the result with the patient.

5.7.2 Explaining the diagnosis

We will discuss explaining things to patients generally in this section since in some of the cases you meet you might well be given the diagnosis in the form of an investigation result or an entry in the patient's clinical record. There are two important principles in explaining things to patients in a patient-centred way:

- Tailoring the explanation to the individual patient
- Checking that the patient has understood your explanation.

Tailoring the explanation means not only that you pitch your explanation at an appropriate level for the patient and use language the patient can easily understand, but also that you must take into account their previous knowledge and health beliefs. The starting point should generally be to check what the patient knows already (or thinks they know). This raises the same issues as establishing their thoughts about what might be wrong in the first place, so a direct approach, for example asking something like: '*What do you know about angina?*' might not elicit much, whereas asking: '*Had you heard of angina?*' will generally elicit a positive response, following which you can ask: '*What sort of things had you heard about it?*'.

Much of what you ask and explain to the patient will depend on your patient's intellectual and educational level — a question that might be worded appropriately for an unskilled factory worker might appear patronising to a university lecturer. Even so you should avoid making too many assumptions; sometimes an apparently poorly educated patient might surprise you with their knowledge, and some highly educated patients may have huge knowledge gaps. It goes without saying that you should use language your patient can understand and avoid using jargon.

Experience of watching GP registrars consulting on video is not terribly reassuring! Unfortunately it seems doctors actually use much more jargon than they think they are using. Watch some videos of yourself consulting with the specific remit of jargon-spotting. Once you become aware of the problem it is not difficult to keep it in mind while consulting and adjust your language accordingly. The reasons doctors use jargon is because often the jargon allows us to define or describe something much more concisely or accurately. Part of the problem lies in the fact that patients do not often give us the right sort of feedback — when we tell them something they do not understand they will often collude and act as if they understand exactly what you mean, generally to avoid making themselves or yourself appear stupid.

Checking that the patient has understood your explanation is probably something you find quite difficult. Certainly it seems to cause candidates a lot of problems in the old style MRCGP video. Candidates in the MRCGP video tried two approaches that generally fell flat with the patients and caused the examiners considerable irritation, so are best avoided. The first is to ask the patient to repeat back to you what you have just explained to them. While this approach does sometimes work it more often than not makes the patient feel very uncomfortable and results in a rather dysfunctional consultation. The second is to ask the patient what they are going to tell their husband or wife when they get home. Again, it does sometimes work but it often causes patients consternation as it is not a question they are expecting. They are also not quite sure why you are asking them since it is not obvious to all of them that what you are doing is checking understanding. One of the most amusing responses I have heard was: '*I won't be telling her anything, because it's none of her business*', which certainly brought home the issue of confidentiality to that candidate!

Sometimes just asking simply: '*Is all that clear to you?*', or '*Is there any of that you'd like me to go over again?*' can be sufficient. However in some cases this is simply not going to be enough.

Make it seem as if it is quite natural not to understand everything by making it clear that medical things are quite complex and difficult to understand, and also by the same token that they are quite difficult for us to explain clearly. So you might say something such as: '*Most patients find that difficult to understand first time round, would you like me to go over some of it again?*', or '*I'm aware that's a lot to take in ...*' or, '*There's lots of information there, does it all make sense?'*. You must deliver it in a way that encourages the patient to believe that you really do expect a response. You can make it seem like you think it might be your own fault if they do not understand it by using phrases such as: *'I often find it difficult to get that across clearly, did that make sense to you?'*, or *'I'm not sure I explained that very well...'*.

If what you are explaining really is quite complex, it might be worth breaking it into smaller, more manageable portions and checking understanding as you go along. It is also often helpful to offer to see the patient again to go over any bits they do not understand; of course you cannot see the patient again in the clinical skills assessment but if the offer is delivered credibly the examiner is likely to give you credit for it.

Information leaflets

Many doctors use information leaflets — many of the clinical software systems incorporate them, or you can use Prodigy. Of course none of these will be available to you during your consultations in the clinical skills assessment, but you can offer a leaflet to the patient. Do not use leaflets as an alternative to explaining things properly though. It is sometimes helpful to just write the diagnosis down on a piece of paper and suggest the patient look it up for themselves and suggest resources they can use on the Internet. Offer to discuss or explain what they find when they come back to see you again.

5.7.3 Formulating a management plan

Once you have made a diagnosis and explained it to the patient you need to do something about it. In any consultation you will have various options available to you, and it is important that you think about this carefully. It often works as a sort of cascade, moving from the most minimal interventions through to the more significant ones.

The first option available to you is to do nothing. While it can often be applied quite literally, it generally involves doing nothing more than explaining things to the patient or reassuring them and allowing some time.

The next step up the ladder is to actually provide some treatment by prescribing. If this is not going to solve the problem you may need to refer the patient to a specialist or to another team member.

Sometimes hospital admission is appropriate. I will discuss each of these steps in the next few sections.

Prescribing

Before discussing what to prescribe we need to discuss the decision whether or not to prescribe at all. It is often stated that the first ethical principle is to do no harm and although it is possible to have done some harm by this stage in the consultation the risks start to get much higher as soon as you reach for the prescription pad. Doctors (and many patients) often overestimate the benefits of drugs and underestimate the side effects. Offering the patient a prescription immediately medicalises the problem, with implications in terms of how seriously the patient perceives the problem both now and for the future, with knock-on effects on future help-seeking behaviour.

Sometimes you can recommend an over-the-counter treatment that can be bought without a prescription. This does to some extent reduce the medicalisation and will not require you to see the patient to issue prescriptions if the problem recurs, but the issues are the same with respect to the ratio between benefit and risk.

In the clinical skills assessment you will be provided with some dummy FP10 prescriptions which will look almost identical to the prescriptions used by an NHS GP. Do not worry too much about putting all the patient's details on there — the patient's name is enough. The drug name and dose are however important, as may be the quantity. Use the drug's generic name rather than the proprietary one unless there is a good reason to (there are certain drugs that should be prescribed by proprietary name, usually controlled release drugs or those where bioavailability varies between preparations). In fact you often do not need to physically hand over a prescription at all, what the examiner is interested in is your prescribing decision-making, so in most cases an explanation to the patient of the drug you plan to prescribe them along with the dosage instructions will suffice.

Choose your drug carefully. Some registrars seem to throw evidence-based medicine out of the window when they think it is mainly consulting skills being tested, but the clinical skills assessment is a test of your clinical skills and the examiners will be keen to see that you prescribe appropriately. You need to get into the habit of thinking explicitly about why you prescribe the drugs you do. Whenever you prescribe in your normal surgeries get into the habit of thinking about how you would justify each prescription to your trainer if he were to ask you to. Ask yourself the following questions:

- What are the particular features of the drug you are prescribing?
- Why is this drug better than the alternatives?
- Are there any specific guidelines for the condition you are treating?
- How many tablets should you prescribe?
- Are there any safety issues such as risk of overdose?
- Are there any interactions with the patient's existing medication?

When you have made your choice you need to make sure you give the patient information about the drug you have prescribed, and this includes how and when it should be taken and any side effects to expect. You should also check that this has been understood and see if the patient has any questions about it.

Dealing with prescription requests

It is possible that you might see a patient where issuing a prescription is the main focus of the consultation, for example where a patient is asking for a specific drug to be prescribed, or where the patient has seen a consultant or other colleague who is recommending a particular treatment. It is likely in this case that the drug will be something you might not feel terribly comfortable prescribing. This might be because it is a drug you do not know enough about, an 'alternative' therapy, a very expensive drug, or one that is not actually licensed for the condition the patient has.

While it might seem that the challenge in these cases is how much you actually know about the drug, in reality the 'nub' of the case is likely to centre on the negotiation with the patient, how well you manage to set out the advantages and disadvantages of prescribing the drug and negotiate a mutually acceptable way forward. There is an element of honesty involved and you should be prepared to set out the reasons for your reticence clearly but sensitively to the patient. Do not forget that while you might be able to pull the wool over the patient's eyes the examiner will not be fooled by spurious rules or guidelines that prevent you prescribing it, so only refer to guidelines that really exist and make sure you recall them accurately.

Think about what negotiation actually means — it does not mean just saying no! It generally means that there is a constructive dialogue between the two parties. It is important to find out as much as you can about why the patient thinks the treatment might be helpful and try not to be dismissive. Your decision will need to be based on a balance between doing good (beneficence), not doing harm (non-maleficence), the patient's autonomy, and the broader implications for the NHS (distributive justice) in the case of a very expensive drug.

If you do decide the requested drug is not something you are prepared to prescribe (and of course sometimes it is right for a doctor to say no), you will then need to be able to justify this to the patient and be able to offer the patient some other way forward.

In today's society patient autonomy carries a lot of weight. This is quite rightly so, but while a patient has a right to choose a treatment that might have potential for harm, do not forget that you as a professional also have autonomy and the right to decline to be party to that treatment. If society intended patients to have total autonomy over what drugs they take we would not have a 'prescription only' category for drugs. The examiners will want you to facilitate the patient making an informed choice but a line has to be drawn somewhere.

Referral

You may come across a patient in the clinical skills assessment who requires a referral. This referral may be to any other health professional, for example to someone else within your primary health care team (physiotherapist, counsellor), a local consultant or even as an emergency admission. For the purposes of the assessment you should assume you are working in a 'normal' NHS general practice with the usual array of facilities and team members and with a district general hospital available. It is probably easiest for you to imagine yourself back in your own practice, and to consider the facilities you have available there.

Do not be tempted to offer a referral as an easy way out of what you perceive to be a tricky problem, and this applies to in-house referrals as well as those to secondary care. If the problem is one that the examiners feel you should manage within the consultation or within primary care you will be penalised for failing to do that. It may well be that the patient might give you some hints about this, but beware the patient who is a 'denier' and does not want to go to hospital despite having a potentially life-threatening condition!

If you do offer a referral, the patient may well ask you how long it is likely to be before they receive an appointment. Make sure that you are realistic in any estimates you give — it might be tempting to reassure them that they will be seen in neurology outpatients in a couple of weeks for their headaches, but the examiner is likely to take a dim view of such 'white lies'. A long wait may result in the patient putting you under pressure to come up with an alternative management plan.

If it is the patient who is requesting the referral, approach the request as you would with a prescription demand as discussed previously. Do not overlook the negative aspects of a referral: not only are there resource implications, getting onto the hospital conveyor belt can have negative implications for patients in terms of over-medicalisation and unpleasant investigations. You should always explore whether the problem might be better dealt with in primary care or using other resources.

5.7.4 Involving the patient
When considering your management plan you should ensure that you involve the patient in the decision-making. This particular aspect of consulting skills was one of the more challenging parts of the MRCGP video exam, partly because it is genuinely quite challenging to do well, but also because many candidates looked like they were attempting it in their video consultations without having really practised it much. As a consequence their attempts often looked a little wooden and contrived. Many seemed to take the literal wording of the exam's performance criterion which used the term 'sharing management options' without really considering why it was there and what it really meant. It is far better to think in terms of 'involving the patient' in management decisions, establishing their preferences regarding treatment and taking those into consideration appropriately.

Of course there are times when things are fairly clear-cut and there is only one appropriate course of action, or where some of the management options are inappropriate for various reasons. It has already been pointed out that being patient-centred does not simply mean doing what the patient wants. For example if faced with a patient presenting with a serious or life-threatening condition whose initial approach is to deny the problem you probably need to spend some time persuading them to accept appropriate management. Similarly, you should not offer inappropriate management options, for example antibiotics, for a patient with a self-limiting upper respiratory infection.

The first step in involving the patient is to define what management options are appropriate and available to you. First of all think carefully about whether you really do need to do anything or if a 'wait and see' approach is reasonable. Factors to consider include the likelihood of a bad outcome if you do not do something, and the likely benefit of any treatment you might offer balanced by the potential harm of the treatment.

Establish the individual patient's personal preferences; some patients are generally averse to taking tablets and would rather tolerate symptoms than resort to medication, while others have a 'pill for every ill' mindset. Some patients are fairly fatalistic and may prefer not to be terribly interventionist, while others will want to investigate every symptom and leave no stone unturned in a quest for symptom control or risk reduction. Some patients prefer the more old-fashioned treatments, while others have faith in new technology. Some patients have a pathological fear of hospitals and investigations. Preferences may well be volunteered but otherwise it is your job to discover them.

Patients' previous experiences, or those of their friends and family, may have a bearing on their preferences. For example, a patient who knows a relative who has had a serious operative complication will not be reassured by the statistic that show that it happens in less than 1 in 1000 cases. The way the media presents risk also influences patients — for example parents are terrified of their child dying of meningitis even though the absolute risk is low (Edwards et al, 2002; Elwyn et al, 1999). Consider the case scenarios below:

Case scenario: Inguinal hernia

A patient presents with an inguinal hernia.

Doctor-centred approach: referral to a surgeon.

Patient-centred approach: Consider this patient's risks of developing problems if the hernia is left untreated. Assess any other ongoing medical problems that impinge on their anaesthetic risk. Asses other physical factors: is the hernia actually giving the patient any trouble? Are there age and mobility factors? Consider the status of the patient: a young fit manual worker would undoubtedly see this differently compared to an elderly diabetic. Do not make any assumptions.

> ### Case scenario: Raised blood pressure
>
> **How do you treat a patient who has had a series of three blood pressure readings over the previous few months, all just above the recommended treatment threshold?**
>
> **Doctor-centred approach**: follow guidelines (e.g. NICE) and tell the patient he/she needs treatment.
>
> **Patient-centred approach**: make a more customised risk-assessment for the patient and try to help them understand the risks and benefits. In reality unless you have a particularly high-risk patient the absolute benefit of drug treatment is fairly low, with high number needed to treat (NNTs). Some patients will want to get onto treatment as soon as possible whereas others might prefer to explore other non-medical approaches through diet and exercise, etc.

5.8 Challenging scenarios

This section will cover some 'set pieces' of the clinical skills assessment — those scenarios that are very likely to turn up in one guise or another. You will experience a wide variety of clinical scenarios when you sit the assessment, but there are certain to be some recurring themes. Although the scenarios may change from one sitting of an exam to another (the patient's name, age and sex, the actual condition), the issues to be dealt with in many of the consultations will recur. In this section I will present some 'generic' issues that are likely to occur and discuss how you should attempt to deal with them.

First of all though, a 'warning'. Use this section to prepare you for what to expect but do not take any of these example too literally; they are here to give you some examples and to demonstrate how some of the problems are generalisable as are the skills you use to tackle them. I will refer to the risks of trying to 'learn' cases in the section on pitfalls later on. The scenarios described below are not based on any knowledge of the actual clinical skills assessment case bank, they are derived from reflection on what skills the examiners would like to test that can feasibly be tested in the clinical skills assessment format. If you keep a diary of the cases you see in a typical week in general practice and grade them in terms of challenge, you will probably find lots of these appear in that list. You might identify some others yourself.

5.8.1 Breaking bad news
This is probably one of the more challenging scenarios. There are lots of

possible clinical scenarios, but the main point of the case is the same: you will be imparting some bad news to the patient.

This will generally be fairly obvious and you are likely to be given a result in the form of a straight test result such as an X-ray, scan, or blood test, or possibly a letter from a consultant. The diagnosis could be a malignancy, but there are other possibilities like neurological disorders such as multiple sclerosis or motor neurone disease. You may well be given the diagnosis in the patient notes, so you may have a couple of minutes before the patient comes in to gather your thoughts and do a little planning. There is not likely to be much preamble in the consultation as the examiners will want you to get to the main issue quickly — ten minutes is not a long time to deal with it.

Your first thoughts might be about the actual condition itself. You must reassure yourself that you are not expected to have specialist knowledge of the condition. Of course you do need some factual knowledge, but by the time you sit this exam you are likely to have been a qualified doctor for at least three years and you will have had at least six months experience in general practice, so you are not likely to encounter anything that completely flummoxes you. Remind yourself that a case like this is designed primarily to test your communication skills and your empathy.

The first principle in breaking bad news is choosing a time and place, but of course this is all outside your control in the assessment! You can make sure you are seated close to the patient without a desk intervening between you. The patient's opening statement is likely to be something such as: '*I've come for my test results doctor*', or '*You asked me to come and see you*'.

Find out what the patient knows or suspects already. You can do this by asking the patient what their understanding of the purpose of the test was, or to ask them to recap their main symptoms and establish what they think might be wrong using the techniques we discussed earlier in this chapter. Do not however spend too long on this: a patient expecting an important result may become frustrated if you make them wait too long for the information and you have quite a lot to try to get done in only ten minutes.

Prepare the patient

What you do next will depend on whether the patient indicates that they suspect something serious or not. If they do not seem to suspect something serious then it is generally recommended that you give them warning early on that you have bad news for them. There is a balance to be struck — you need to be open, honest and direct but at the same time to deliver the information sensitively and not be too direct initially. You could say something such as: '*Well I'm sorry but the test results are quite serious*', or '*I'm afraid I have some bad news for you*'. You then need to pause to let it sink in and give the patient a chance to respond. As always you need to respond appropriately to the patient's reaction and it is no good learning set phrases for this.

If the patient still gives no indication of any specific suspicions you need to give them the news, preferably slowly, a bit at a time and using language they will understand. If the patient does seem to have suspicions you ought to establish what those suspicions are and confirm the diagnosis for them, again taking time and not giving too much information at once.

In the clinical skills assessment your patient is likely to be alone, but it is worth asking at this stage if they would prefer to have someone with them, and offer to contact a partner or friend. You might also like to ask if they would prefer to defer further discussion until they can come back with someone.

Use of language

When discussing the diagnosis language is of course vitally important. Giving patients serious diagnoses is an unpleasant task and is often difficult emotionally for the doctor too. All too often this leads doctors to use slightly vague terms or ones which are a bit ambiguous, talking about 'shadows' on chest X-rays, or a 'mass' in the abdomen. The terms 'benign' and 'malignant' have very clear meaning to us as doctors but probably not to most patients. What patients want to know is whether they have cancer or not, and it is best not to avoid this issue and to actually use the word 'cancer' since it removes any ambiguity completely. You really must take time to check that the patient understands what you are telling them, and to ask them if they have any questions.

Patient reaction

Patients will react in many different ways; they can be upset and tearful, or simply go very quiet and reflective. Some may even be angry, particularly if there has been any delay in the diagnosis. You must respond appropriately and with empathy. This may involve silence on your part, using touch such as placing a hand on the patient's arm or verbal expressions such as: '*I'm sorry, I know this is really difficult for you*'. Simply acknowledging their reaction can be useful, for example: '*I can see that you're quite shocked/angry*'. It might be worth checking again if they would prefer you to contact someone to accompany them.

Most patients will want to know something about what treatment can be offered and their prognosis. As a GP you may well feel unable to be too specific about this, and most patients will be referred on to specialist care, but it is important that you do attempt to give them some indications as to what sort of treatment to expect. It is important to emphasise that you will be able to do something, to give the patient some hope, but without being inappropriately optimistic. Giving prognoses is fraught with problems and is generally best avoided, especially in the initial stages.

Your patient will want to know what is going to happen next and it is important that you are very specific and very clear about this. If their diagnosis is one of cancer, or potentially so, make them aware of the specific rules within the NHS for managing this, for example the 'two-week rule'. Reassure them that they will be prioritised and that you will make sure they are seen quickly.

At times like these patients need to feel supported and like to know exactly what is going to happen and who to contact. This is a time when a GP taking personal responsibility really does help, so it is important that you stress your availability to the patient and let them know how they can contact you. It might be helpful to arrange a specific time for them to come back so you can clarify any questions they might have, to see them with a partner or close relative if they would like that, and to let them know how you are progressing with their referral.

If the patient is distraught think about asking if they would like a quiet room to sit in to recover, and ask if someone can come to collect them if they came alone.

A consultation where you are breaking bad news is likely to be emotionally draining (you may be shocked at how well the role-players can play such roles!). During your normal surgeries you can take a bit of time out after a difficult consultation (deal with a couple of phone calls or grab a cup of coffee), but you cannot do this in the clinical skills assessment and your next patient is only a couple of minutes away. Move on mentally and emotionally as soon as the patient has left the room. Do not sit there dwelling on how well or badly you think you handled the consultation; get on with reading the notes for your next patient and start to gather your thoughts about how you are going to tackle the next consultation.

5.8.2 Consultations with children

You may have a consultation with a child in the clinical skills assessment, and if so it is likely they will be accompanied by a parent or guardian. Do not lose sight of who your patient is — in reality it is both of them although the child is of course the prime consideration. See my earlier comments regarding current (lack of) use of child role-players in the assessment – there are however no reasons actually stopping the examiners introducing them, and they were successfully used in the previous MRCGP simulated surgery assessment.

Although the parent is likely to do a lot of the talking you really must do your best to engage with the child at an appropriate level. That means putting them at their ease by being relaxed and friendly, facing the child and maintaining eye contact with them while asking questions rather than looking at the parent. If the parent answers your questions anyway (as they often tend to do), you can still try to involve the child by seeking confirmation or further clarification of the parent's answers. Obviously much of this will depend on the age and maturity of the child, but in reality presenting you with very young children in the clinical skills assessment is unlikely as the child will have to be old enough to understand the role and the sort of responses they will be expected to provide.

Confidentiality and consent

If you think the child is mature enough you may feel it useful to have a chat to them alone. This can be tricky to put to the parent(s), but if phrased appropriately most parents will understand. You need to ask also if the child is happy to have a chat alone. It might be important to explain to an older child the issues around confidentiality, as most will be unaware that you have a duty to respect their confidentiality. It can facilitate the conversation if you reassure them that before the parent comes back into the room the two of you will agree what is divulged. Whatever their maturity remember that a child is unlikely to divulge information regarding drug or alcohol use, sexual activity and contraception with a parent present.

The legalities around consent and confidentiality are complex and not always intuitive. With older children the issue of competence arises — you may have heard of the phrases 'Gillick competence' and 'Fraser competence', referring to the names involved in the famous legal case that set precedent. Is this child mature enough to be able to make their own decisions and take responsibility for themselves? There is no quick and easy way of doing this, in reality most of our assessments are subconscious as we take in the patient's general demeanour and use of language, but you must make sure you explicitly check their understanding of the issues raised in the consultation, again being mindful not to patronise.

You can get information from the parent too; they will probably have an opinion about whether the child is able to decide things for themselves. Your problem arises when you think the child is competent but the parent wants to make the decisions!

When it comes to negotiating management plans the ideal situation is to keep both parent and child happy, but again the child is the more important of the two. You really must involve both in the discussion.

In the case of a parent presenting without the child being present you may feel that it is important that you arrange to actually see the child face to face but you should be flexible about this — a straight refusal to discuss the issue is likely to anger the patient and not do your grading on the case any good! While it is generally good practice to arrange to see the child at a later date the case will generally be written such that you can make some progress with the problem in the child's absence.

5.8.3 Cultural issues

Language may be one obvious barrier — engaging in the subtleties of the consulting skills we have discussed is a whole new ball game if it has to be done via an interpreter (whether the interpreter is present in the room or whether they are on the end of the phone as in when you use Language Line).

Some cultures may be much more deferential to a doctor and might expect a much more doctor-centred approach than you have been encouraged to utilise. Even non-verbal communication can be confusing — avoiding eye contact may indicate respect rather than embarrassment, for example.

Different cultures will have different attitudes towards medicine, with many being far more likely to expect a more medicalising approach than we are used to in the UK.

Muslim women may not wish to be uncovered for a clinical examination, so it is even more important to sensitively ask permission to examine and be prepared to compromise; a slightly inadequate examination through clothes may well be better than no examination at all, but be prepared to be a little more persuasive if there is a potentially serious problem.

The clinical skills assessment is not a test of your factual knowledge of the cultural differences between various ethnic groups, so do not worry that you are not aware of a specific ethnic group's health belief tendencies, etc. just be aware that any patient you meet might have a different set of values and beliefs to yourself and that you should make no assumptions, instead making an explicit effort to sensitively explore them.

5.8.4 An angry patient

Dealing with anger is a challenging skill, and in the context of a consultation even more so since the patient's anger will often arise from a potential shortcoming on our own part or of a colleague.

Patients get angry for all sorts of reasons, sometimes because they think we have made an error or not helped them as much as they would have liked, but sometimes because they think a colleague of ours has let them down. Sometimes it can just be from frustration that medicine in general is unable to help them, or because of shortcomings of the system within the NHS (for example a long waiting list or a rationed treatment).

Of course the principles of managing an angry patient or even one who is just unhappy are similar no matter what the cause. We often need to curtail our natural reactions, which are generally to be angry back or to run and take cover!

The first thing is to try to remain calm yourself and concentrate on the skills you are going to use to manage the situation. Your active listening skills are important in these cases, so make it obvious to the patient that you are listening and that you are interested in hearing what they have to say.

Acknowledging their feelings is important. Try saying something such as: '*I can see you're pretty angry about this...*', or '*This has clearly upset you*'.

Use the skills we have discussed earlier to establish exactly what the patient is angry about and what their expectations of you are. You need to establish all the facts so you have got a clear idea of what has happened, summarising it back to the patient to make sure you have understood correctly. You can do all this without actually expressing any opinion, and you should try to remain neutral — we naturally find this difficult if the patient is blaming us for something or if they are blaming a colleague, as doctors we generally have a natural loyalty to our partners, staff, even the local systems in which we work. It can be helpful to explain to a patient that in order to try to help them you would like to run through exactly what has happened. Allowing the patient to feel that someone has listened to their account of what has happened can in itself defuse the situation.

You do not need to admit fault on anyone's behalf at this stage; a statement such as: '*I can see why that would upset you*' expresses understanding and empathy for their emotion without accepting any blame.

Once you have completed your information gathering you can start to analyse the situation. Sometimes you might think the patient is being completely unreasonable, and at others you might well agree that they have been hard done by, but you should attempt to remain neutral. No matter what the patient tells you it is more than likely that you will need to get information from elsewhere to corroborate or triangulate, and you should sensitively explain this to them. If the patient is made to feel that you are taking their concerns seriously and that you will look into the situation it is likely they will be calmer and be happy to work with you constructively to solve the problem.

As has already been mentioned, when a patient confronts us with anger a natural response is to be defensive with all the associated body language that goes with it. Be aware of this and concentrate on trying to remain relaxed with an open posture and try to establish rapport. Role-players consistently report that they find it very difficult maintaining the anger when they are faced with a doctor who is being skilfully disarming!

Making a complaint

What you should not do is either behave very defensively or collude with the patient in criticising a colleague. Being defensive will make them feel you are not going to help them, and criticising a colleague is potentially unprofessional. If you think a colleague (or even you yourself) has behaved or acted inappropriately, it might be acceptable to say that it does look like that may be possible, but that you will need to establish more information and hear the colleague's side of the story first. If the patient is unhappy about a colleague within the practice it might be appropriate to offer to arrange to meet them with the patient. If there is potential for a complaint you should facilitate this and explain how to go about this constructively.

You must be aware of and be able to explain to the patient the procedures for making a complaint. Although these will vary slightly from practice to practice they are generally very similar and the best approach is probably to stick with the procedures that apply in your own practice.

Of course sometimes patients really are downright unreasonable and if so you will need to address this at some stage; if the patient has unrealistic expectations of what a doctor or staff member can do, of what medicine in general can do or of what the NHS can reasonably provide, then you might need to attempt to sensitively manage those expectations.

There might be scope for you to do something to put the situation right, for example in arranging or expediting a hospital appointment, or in providing appropriate treatment yourself. You should say that you will do what you can to put the situation right to the patient's satisfaction, but beware making it seem that you are doing this to distract from dealing with the cause of the patient's emotion.

Make sure the consultation ends with an agreed plan of action with a definite timescale. Let the patient know you will be happy to speak to them again as taking personal responsibility and providing continuity is important.

5.8.5 A disabled patient

Patients present with all sorts of disability, but clearly within the context of the clinical skills assessment there is a limit on what you might meet. It might be as simple as a patient with a walking stick or crutches, but you may encounter a blind or deaf patient.

Acknowledge the disability rather than pretend it is not there, and think of ways you can help the patient. Try to imagine being that patient and what effect the disability might have on coming to see a doctor. The patient might need to be guided to a chair for example, or you might need to move your chair to accommodate a wheelchair. You might have a patient who is partially deaf where you need to speak loudly and clearly, on the other hand they may be profoundly deaf meaning you need to either use a sign language interpreter or communicate by writing.

Make sure you continue to take the disability into consideration throughout the consultation, and ask yourself if the patient needs any help from you (for example in undressing or getting dressed again). Consider the disability in formulating and negotiating your management plan — do not make assumptions about what the patient can or cannot do, and ask them if they think they will be able to manage. Disabled patients do not like being patronised, and those with long-term disabilities are often more capable than we would imagine. They also know how best an able-bodied person is able to help them so don't be afraid to ask.

5.8.6 Hidden agendas

A hidden agenda is when a patient presents with a problem but the actual main problem is not the presenting complaint. Sometimes the presenting complaint can be a complete red herring, in which case it is sometimes referred to as a token presentation. Patients do this for a couple of reasons. Often because they are worried you will think they are neurotic, or because they are embarrassed or ashamed about the problem they have, or sometimes because they are in a form of denial. In this case they might 'check you out' with something fairly innocuous, and if they find you sympathetic and consider they can trust you they may then divulge the real problem that is on their mind. At other times the presenting complaint is the main problem but there is some hidden fear or anxiety that you have to work at uncovering.

How do you know if there might be a hidden agenda? It can be very difficult, but the key thing is to gain the patient's trust by being empathic and a good listener. Sometimes there will be cues or hints that there is something else on their mind, for example pauses, failure to maintain eye contact or generally looking uncomfortable.

In the clinical skills assessment the patient is likely to give you more of a chance than in 'real life', and they will be consciously giving you cues. However the actors are very well trained and highly skilled and if you do not establish good rapport and you do not make them feel they trust you they will withhold cues.

If you suspect there is something else on the patient's mind you should probe carefully, acknowledging the signs you have identified, for example by saying *'You're looking worried'*, or *'You seem as if there's something else on your mind'*. Be prepared to use silence, and if you still think there is something else you can ask directly if there is anything they are worried about. They will not deliberately mislead you and if you directly ask if there is anything else on their mind they will give you some form of clue that there is a hidden agenda. Sometimes you might be able to second guess what it is as we discussed previously. A key piece of advice is to trust the patient and take a denial of any other worries at face value. There seems to be an assumption amongst the GP training community that the majority of clinical skills assessment cases will have a hidden agenda. This is not the case and you can waste valuable time if you keep probing for a problem that simply is not there!

When you think you know what is going on it is useful again to summarise it back to check that you are grasping the issues correctly. Do not forget the problem they originally presented with; it is worth checking if this is something they would still like dealt with or whether it was in fact fairly unimportant to them.

5.8.7 Psychosocial problems

A high proportion of the patients we see in general practice are presenting with problems that have a psychosocial basis and this will be reflected in the clinical skills assessment.

You could be presented with a patient with depression, anxiety, phobia, obsessive compulsive disorder or any other psychiatric conditions. Patients sometimes present to us with distress resulting from their social circumstances, and it is important that you are able to explore these appropriately and differentiate between what is a social problem and what is an illness. For example not all patients who are unhappy are actually depressed. There are two issues in these consultations:

- Identifying psychological illness
- Putting patients problems into a psychosocial context

Diagnosing psychological illness is like diagnosing any other illness; you take a history, encouraging the patient to tell you their story, and find out what they think about the problem (as we have discussed already). Then you must conduct an examination, in this case not a physical one but a psychological one. It is important that you ask all the right questions to explore their illness fully — by the time you get this far you should have a good idea of what the problem is and therefore tailor your questions appropriately.

Assess severity

You need to establish the severity of the illness; if you have a depressed patient it is really important that you establish the degree of risk of self-harm. This should have been done to death in your teaching sessions with your trainer, but do not forget it in the exam! There are various ways of doing this, from asking directly if they have actually considered suicide (which can sometimes be appropriate) to the more subtle: *'Have you ever felt so low that you've considered hurting yourself?'*. We all see patients who say they are suicidal but actually are not, so if they do express suicidal thoughts you need to check this out by perhaps asking things such as how they thought they might do it or what has stopped them from doing it.

Similarly, if you have a patient who says they are hearing voices you need to find out how often it happens, what sort of things the voices say and how distressing they find it. If you think you have a psychotic patient you then must explore whether they represent a risk to others.

Social context

The other issue is to put the patient's problems into a social context. Whether the problem is physical or psychological you must explore the social aspects, and there is so much more to this than merely asking what they do for a living, whether they are married or how many children they have. By all means ask what their job is, but even more importantly, how does their illness affect their ability to do it? Is the illness affecting their relationships at home, what does the patient's wife/husband/ partner think about the problem? Does it affect their hobbies?

Consider how medical conditions might affect your own lifestyle — what if it prevented you from driving, playing golf, tennis, etc? How would you feel about that?

5.8.8 Third parties

You will probably recognise that we often have a third party involved in a consultation, either because they come with the patient but sometimes because they come on a patient's behalf. For example, consider a patient attending with a friend or relative. You need to consider why the third party is there. The obvious answer is that they are there at the patient's request to give some moral support, but do not make assumptions! Very often the patient might say: *'I hope you don't mind my partner coming in with me?'*, in which case at least you know who the other person is and the implication then is that they are there with the patient's consent. On the other hand the other person might say something such as: *'I'm John's wife, do you mind if I come in with him?'*, in which case you might be left wondering whose idea it was that she attend with him, or indeed whose idea it was that he come to the doctor in the first place!

In each of these scenarios you are given the opportunity to check that your patient is happy to be accompanied — for the latter you might say something like: *'You're very welcome so long as John doesn't mind'*. If there is no introduction it is reasonable to ask who the other person is, and to ask the patient if they would rather consult you with them present or if they would rather see you alone.

Remember that while the other person might be there with good intentions, and while you do not want to offend them, your first duty is to the patient, and you must always bear in mind that it may be that they would rather see you on their own, at least for some of the consultation.

Even if the third party is there at the patient's request the consultation may stray into personal or sensitive areas that might lead you to suspect that their continued presence could be inhibitory, in which case it is your job to suggest that perhaps it would be helpful to have a chat with the patient alone. Sometimes patients are genuinely nervous about coming to the doctor and do appreciate the support of a friend or relative accompanying them, but once they are there it is likely that your communication skills will put them at ease so that they no longer need them there.

Sometimes the third party will speak for the patient, in which case it is generally best to thank them for trying to help but to gently say that you find it more useful to hear it in the patient's own words. They may even try to take charge of the consultation, which makes it a little more difficult. In this case try to see if you can get by with a little diplomacy and prompting the patient, but if it is becoming disruptive it is best to take charge and ask if you could have a moment with the patient alone.

A third party presenting without the patient

Next we need to consider the third party presenting without the patient. If this is a parent presenting on behalf of a child then it makes life easier in that confidentiality is less of an issue, especially for younger children.

In the case of a presumably competent adult it is more difficult. It is important to let the person know that you do appreciate their concern but to gently remind them that you cannot really have much of a two-way conversation since you cannot discuss the patient's medical issues without consent. A common scenario is a son or daughter expressing concern about an elderly parent. You need to remember the rules of confidentiality which are that you cannot breach it unless (in this scenario) you have the patient's explicit consent or you are fully confident that the breach is in the patient's best interests. It is fine to gather information from the relative but with the understanding that it is a one-way conversation. Sometimes relatives make it more difficult for you by asking you not to disclose the conversation to the patient, and although this can sometimes be justified, you must proceed with caution. Lay people generally underestimate the confidentiality issues and often fail to see the pitfalls in a deception, but it is often very difficult to avoid the deception being uncovered — which can have disastrous consequences for the doctor/patient relationship. It may be possible for you to give some generic advice without actually discussing any of the patient's medical details. If you feel you can help the patient without breaching confidentiality then do so as a flat refusal to help until the patient comes to see you is generally inappropriate.

Another common scenario you may recognise is that of a relative not wanting a patient to be told the full extend of the truth about a terminal diagnosis, which does of course beg the question how they knew about it before the patient in the first place! In this case it is almost never appropriate to collude with the request, you must discuss the situation with the patient themselves and come to your own conclusion about how much it is appropriate to tell them. Of course you will need to explain carefully to the relative the rules under which you must operate as a doctor and explain why it is a bad idea to lie to your patient.

Health professionals consulting about a patient

A similar but slightly different scenario is when another health professional consults about a patient. This is quite different in that if this is someone who is involved in providing care for the patient you do have the right to discuss confidential medical information with them.

In this context what you must do is consider the different roles the two of you have in providing care for the patient and how you can work synergistically to maximise team-working and enhance the care provided. Try to consider the specific skills each of you brings to the partnership, clarify exactly why the other professional has approached you and find out what they thought you might do - in some ways you must continue to use the same communication skills as with a patient, that is find out what the other health professional's ideas, concerns and expectations are. Consider the information they bring to you and ask yourself what else you need to know before contemplating any action. Perhaps you need to arrange to assess the patient first. Make sure you do not get coerced into something you might later regret!

5.8.9 'Expert' patients

In this section we will consider the issues raised by a patient who has an in-depth knowledge of the medical problem they have, either because they are just generally well-informed and have researched it for themselves, or perhaps they themselves have a medical qualification. Doctors may often find this sort of scenario quite threatening — we are worried they might know more than us and expose inadequate knowledge on our part, or perhaps the patients come with very specific ideas and expectations that might not match what we consider to be appropriate.

Another issue is that we must not make assumptions — it is easy to be seduced by a patient who uses lots of medical jargon into believing they are better informed than they actually are. You must remember that the person in front of you is still your patient and that you are the person with the responsibility for making sure the decisions taken are medically appropriate and that your patient fully understands whatever is going on and is taking well informed decisions. If a patient does start using a few medical words it is always worth explicitly checking their occupation (if you have not already done that) or asking them what they have read about the condition.

On the other hand do not be patronising — it can be a delicate balancing act, and as with any other patient you must explore their understanding and expectations explicitly but you should make sure that you acknowledge and value their expertise.

Equality

You must also bear in mind equality. Equality in this context does not mean treating everyone exactly the same; it means treating people according to their circumstances and their needs but being mindful of the needs of others — the issue of distributive justice.

A doctor who consults you about a medical problem will actually have quite different needs to your average lay person — doctors tend to be infrequent consulters and usually self-manage and self-treat minor problems, sometimes major ones too, and often deny there is anything wrong until quite late on in the course of an illness. By the time a doctor presents with a set of symptoms they are far more likely to have significant pathology than other patients, might have already tried some treatment (either available over the counter or prescription only) and may even have done some investigations. A fellow health professional is also going to be only too aware of the more serious diagnoses in the differential list which is likely to result in them being more worried than the average patient. Therefore it might be quite appropriate to make yourself a little more accessible and to take their concerns a little more seriously. This is not favouritism; it is acknowledging and responding to different needs.

However beware of the colleague or well informed patient who expects you to ignore usual practice or protocols, prescribe inappropriate treatments or refer when it is not necessary. You must always negotiate a management plan that you are comfortable with.

5.9 Safety

As the nMRCGP is a licensing exam for general practice there is a lot of emphasis on safety. Make sure that in your quest for demonstrating your communication skills and patient-centred approach you do not overlook the clinical medicine. In addition to all the active listening and exploring patient agendas you must also take a systematic medical history, conduct a competent clinical examination where appropriate, and make sure that your management plan is in keeping with current accepted evidence-based practice.

5.10 Resource issues

We have already touched on the subject of resource usage and this section is a quick reminder that the clinical skills assessment is about general practice in the UK, and that your consultations should take account of some of the vagaries of working within the NHS. One of the principal restrictions on the way GPs practice is that we work within a system that has limited resources. Some treatments are explicitly rationed, for example treatments for impotence or infertility, while others are much more subtle such as the way waiting lists operate and the guidance we receive on prescribing generally.

It is tempting in consultations to try to keep the patient happy, and you will feel under this pressure within the assessment. Being a GP in the UK however is about balancing the wants and needs of the individual patient in front of us with the broader needs of our practice population.

In some clinical areas there is specific guidance from NICE and you will no doubt have revised many of their treatment guidelines in preparing for the applied knowledge test. It is important that you do not mentally discard that information when you sit the clinical skills assessment, since presenting you with a case that involves negotiating with a patient about a treatment where there is a rationing issue offers the examiners an opportunity to present you with multiple challenges.

Investigations

It is an accepted fact that, on average, less experienced doctors investigate patients more than their experienced colleagues. This is partly because they are more accustomed to coping with uncertainty, partly an awareness of the above mentioned resource issues, but also because they recognise the slightly paradoxical fact that investigating patients increases their anxiety levels and concerns about having a serious diagnosis, even when those investigations are normal. There is a wealth of evidence in the medical literature that clearly demonstrates this and it seems the key is probably good communication, explicitly identifying and addressing the patient's true concerns.

You have no doubt also encountered the problem of requesting a battery of tests that you confidently expect to be normal only to find some minor, inexplicable and probably totally irrelevant abnormalities, or tests that are often too non-specific to be helpful such as an ESR or rheumatoid factor. Only request tests that you think might genuinely shed more light on the problem!

5.11 The Quality and Outcomes Framework

In 2004, GPs in the UK were presented with a new contract which included the 'Quality and Outcomes Framework' generally referred to as QOF. This incentivised GPs to pursue targets in key areas of practice, mainly in the realms of chronic disease management. This has impinged on the day-to-day consultations of GPs as they opportunistically gather the data required to meet the targets and thus boost their income. There are many concerns about the effect of this on everyday practice, not least the way in which it can disrupt the consultation. Most of the guidance in this chapter on consulting with patients has been encouraging you to be patient-centred and to focus on the patient's agenda. The QOF targets tend to push GPs in the opposite direction by encouraging us to address issues other than the ones the patient has presented about, and to practice in a much more disease-centred way.

There is good news for you as you can more or less forget about the QOF during the clinical skills assessment. First of all you will not have a computer system to worry about, so there will be no pop-up prompts to check the patient's blood pressure, etc. Second, the examiners recognise that you have got your hands full dealing with what are generally fairly challenging consultations in the 10 minutes allowed so they really do not expect you to attempt any opportunistic health promotion. For the purpose of the clinical skills assessment do not ask about smoking status, blood pressures, whether the patient has had a smear, etc. unless it is directly relevant to the presenting problem.

5.12 How the cases are marked

The first thing to say in this section is that you should not worry too much about how the questions are marked! This section is here to help you understand the process, hopefully to reassure you and to encourage you to concentrate on addressing the patient's problem rather than trying to second guess what the examiner is looking for, which often results in you wasting your time on unhelpful activity.

The examiners
Each patient you see will be accompanied by an examiner. The examiners are all experienced GPs and all have gone through a rigorous selection process followed by specific training for the clinical skills assessment. In addition to this there is an ongoing training programme and rigorous quality assurance to monitor their performance. Most have been examiners for the old MRCGP assessment, but there are many new recruits, most of whom are experienced GP trainers.

Each examiner will be accompanying a patient for the whole day and will therefore only be marking the one case. This means that the examiners can very reliably 'calibrate' for the case they are watching; they have very in-depth knowledge of the case and will have been involved in a calibration exercise for that case along with their role-player and the other role-players and examiners who are involved in that case for the day. They will have a good idea of all the various permutations of approaches candidates could possibly take with the case and have a very clear idea of the level of performance required to achieve a pass for that case. They will have been provided with any evidence (such as guidelines) that may be pertinent to the case.

Three domains

The examiner will make an overall global decision on your performance in the case deciding whether you have clearly passed or failed it or have been a borderline pass or fail. Although it is a global decision, the marking schedule is subdivided into three domains, and for each of these the examiner will award a clear or borderline pass or fail. The examiner will use these three grades to guide the overall decision, but they are not used in a simplistic mathematical way, so you could still pass the case even if you perform badly in one of the domains, and similarly you could still fail even if you did reasonably well in two of the domains. This may sound a bit vague and unscientific, but a guiding principle in the assessment's development has been to avoid marking by check-list. The reason for this is because marking complex behavioural skills and the problem-solving and integrative skills the examination is designed to test is simply not possible by check-list. One of the criticisms of the 'old' video assessment was that it did seem to result in candidates resorting to using these sort of techniques which produced unnatural, dysfunctional consultations. The College wants to avoid this in the clinical skills assessment and reward the kind of behaviours patients would regard as good doctoring — good communication and clinical skills integrated into natural, flowing consultations. The three domains are:

- Data-gathering, technical and assessment skills
- Clinical management skills
- Interpersonal skills.

The reason these are distilled down from the six areas listed at the start of this chapter is largely down to practicality — to expect an examiner to bear six different areas in mind and grade each individually is expecting a bit too much.

When you start to look at individual consultations you will realise that very few require skills from each of these three domains in equal measure, most will be heavily weighted towards one, although some will of course be fairly relatively equally balanced. That is another reason why a global assessment is an advantage over a check-list system where points are awarded for key elements of the consultation — that would require a complex weighting system whereas experienced examiners can incorporate this sort of weighting into a judgement quite easily and naturally, particularly given a little help from the case writers in spelling out the 'nub' of the case and what it is designed to test.

Global judgements are generally in your favour since they allow the examiner to balance mistakes you make against your overall performance and allow them to factor in any parts of the consultation they thought were particularly good. Examiners generally do not like to fail candidates who perform well overall but who make a couple of non-critical slips. Similarly they do not like to pass candidates whose performance they think is generally poor but who slip in a few key words or phrases that might tick a few boxes on a marking schedule.

The three domains are pretty much self-explanatory, but we will spend a little time expanding on them to make sure you understand them.

5.12.1 Data-gathering, technical and assessment skills

This involves taking an adequate history, conducting an appropriate examination and interpreting the information gathered appropriately. This needs to be done in a systematic way with appropriate identification of key findings. It should also be done efficiently, being selective and making good use of time.

5.12.2 Clinical management skills

This domain refers to your decision-making skills — choosing investigations, formulating a differential diagnosis and coming up with a sensible management plan with appropriate prescribing, referral and care management. Also included is practising safely and holistically, being able to manage complex or multiple problems and encouraging a positive attitude and health promotion.

5.12.3 Interpersonal skills

Here the examiners are looking for your ability to connect with the patient, identifying and exploring their ideas, concerns and expectations. You also need to explain effectively and take your patients views into consideration. Also in here is the 'human' aspect of being a doctor — being understanding, considerate and sympathetic, demonstrating empathy, and being non-judgemental.

On the marking schedule the examiner is provided with a series of phrases that illustrate the positive and negative features within each domain — it must be emphasised that these are not used as a check-list but to illustrate the sort of behaviour being looked for and to remind the examiner of some of the poorer examples of consulting that might appear within the domain.

At the end of the consultation the examiner will have awarded three separate domain grades and will have to decide on a single overall grade. Also on the schedule is space to record feedback — this is not in free text format but instead as a series of statements that represent a range of behaviours from which the examiner makes a selection. These can be fed back to you after the exam.

There are no 'tricks' you can use to fool the examiners. They will assess whatever they see, but will also take note of what does not go on in the consultation. Do not think that by avoiding difficult issues you will avoid potentially making mistakes and therefore losing marks — you will lose marks by avoiding issues, whether that means you just left them out completely or tried to skirt around them by arranging to refer the patient or arranging a follow-up appointment next week so you can look something up or ask a colleague about it in the meantime.

The role-player takes no part in the grading, although the examiner may well confer with them before deciding your grade. They will not ask the role-player what grade they think you should have, but might clarify matters of fact with them to confirm things you said or did not say, or to check on their feelings during the consultation. While an examiner gets a very good idea whether they feel you have adequately addressed the patient's concerns or empathised appropriately they sometimes like to double-check this with the role-player.

The examiner may take a prescription into consideration, but again it is used in a global context to inform the grade rather than contributing a specific mark. As was stated earlier they are not worried about the minor technicalities of checking the patient's name and address are completed correctly, but they will be looking to see that it is an appropriate drug used in the correct dose and that you have given a sensible quantity.

As has already been pointed out, a candidate who is performing well generally but makes a couple of slips is likely to pass a case. You are not expected to be perfect, and even the most expert GP would struggle to perform well against all three domains in a complex case with only 10 minutes in which to do it. However there are times when mistakes are considered too critical. Generally speaking a single mistake is only likely to drag you down into the failing zone if it is a fairly significant one — one which might result in putting a patient at risk for example. This would then be reflected in your grade for the one case only.

Since the examiners are all doctors they are subject to the General Medical Council's duties of a doctor to report a colleague whose clinical performance is at such a low standard as to put patients at risk. This does not generally mean making a single mistake, but would need to be a more systematic pattern of behaviour that caused the examiners significant concern and led them to believe that the doctor was likely to be putting patients at risk in his everyday practice. This is generally only when they have seen very chaotic behaviour, for example not listening to patients, being rude or handling the patient roughly, irrational management, etc.

What is needed to pass?
So, what do you need to do to pass overall? It is all very well deciding that you have passed or failed each of the individual 12 cases, but an overall decision as to whether you have passed or failed the CSA has to be reached. This requires a process known as 'standard setting' which is very complex and requires an evaluation of the approximate 'degree of difficulty' of the cases used in any particular sitting. For this reason the 'number needed to pass' is not set in tablets of stone but for all but one of the sittings in the first two years of the exam you have needed to pass eight of the 12 live cases (i.e. the pilot case is excluded). It is very unlikely to drop as low as seven but it is possible that it could rise to nine.

The pass rate overall for candidates sitting the clinical skills assessment for the first time is just over 80%, and in the mid-60s for those attempting for the second time. These numbers are however quite difficult to interpret since they make no allowance for when in ST3 candidates have sat the assessment, and there is wide variation depending on gender, experience, where you have trained, etc. For example within the above pass rate of 80%, female candidates had a pass rate of 88%, with males much lower at 70%. You are also more likely to pass if your primary medical degree was in a medical school within the UK.

Of course these are the early days of the clinical skills assessment and it may be that as trainers and vocational training scheme programme directors become more familiar with what is required to prepare their trainees for the exam that the pass rate rises.

5.13 Pitfalls and common mistakes

In this section we will point out some of the common errors doctors make during their clinical skills assessment consultations and focus on those that will pull your grade down.

The first of these is being doctor-centred early on in the consultation: interrupting the patient, asking closed questions and missing or ignoring cues. Apart from the fact that this sort of behaviour in itself will attract a lower grade, it reduces the information you get. It will almost always result in the information you get from the patient being inferior in both quantity and quality. The role-players are trained to respond well to a patient-centred doctor who is a good listener and will give you fuller descriptions of symptoms, be more prepared to divulge their concerns and health beliefs and will generally make your life easier.

Examination technique
Many registrars just think of this exam as being one about communication skills and ignore the practical clinical examination skills in both their preparation and during the exam itself. Examiners are generally concerned that there seems to be a decline in clinical skills, possibly related partly to the reduced amount of time young doctors spend with patients these days due to shorter working hours in the junior hospital posts, but also probably to an increased reliance on technology (blood tests, X-rays, ultrasound scans, MRIs and CTs).

Examiners have observed that in the examination many registrars seem to appear to go through the motions of conducting an examination but without appearing to be actively seeking physical signs. For example, it is no good simply placing your stethoscope on the patient's chest in what appear to be the correct places, you need to be actively thinking about what you should be hearing there and about what abnormalities you might expect to find.

A third issue is that already referred to earlier in this chapter of avoiding issues. Do not try to fob the patient off — make sure you really do try to address their concerns. Think carefully before suggesting arranging investigations or a referral: is this a problem you can make progress with by good clinical decision-making? The role-players know what is the most appropriate management for their clinical problem and will probably give you cues if you are following a course that will not reward you well on the marking schedule! If you suggest seeing them again after tests or making a referral and the patient seems a little dissatisfied with this, just think again and double check whether your course of action is really the most appropriate.

Lots of candidates seem to resort to handing the patient an imaginary information leaflet. Whilst this can be a useful strategy it should not be used as an alternative to a good explanation. It is sometimes a tempting strategy to use if you are not entirely sure of the facts about the condition you are dealing with, or if you are not confident of them and are worried about explaining the problem in front of the examiner and getting bits of it wrong, in which case be honest and explain to the patient that you cannot recall all the facts but tell them what you can before resorting to the leaflet. Another reason for using them is to save time — it is much quicker to hand over a leaflet than to spend three or four minutes explaining something to a patient and answering their questions. This again is not generally a good reason, it tends to leave patients feeling like they have been fobbed off; patients would usually rather a doctor explain something than read a leaflet. In any case patients can usually access the information you are giving in the leaflet for themselves via the Internet these days.

Inappropriate questions and/or examinations

Make sure your questioning and examination are focused on the patient's problem. Firstly you are short of time and while a few questions do not cost you much time, lots of the unnecessary examinations will cost you quite a lot of time. Try timing yourself checking a patient's blood pressure in surgery; by the time they get their jacket off, sleeve rolled up, you have measured their blood pressure and communicated the result you will find you will not have much change out of two minutes. That is a big chunk out of your available ten minutes.

Do not waste time asking opportunistic health promotion type questions, and unless it is directly relevant to the patient's problem do not ask about alcohol, smoking, when the patient last had a smear, etc. Apart from wasting time some of the personal lifestyle questions can irritate a patient who perceives the information not to be relevant to their problem and even worse may feel that you are being judgemental about them.

Making the diagnosis explicit

Candidates sometimes initiate a treatment without actually making the diagnosis or the actual reason for the treatment explicit to the patient. If you have not explained it clearly to the patient the examiner might be left wondering too! Do not just imply diagnoses, spell them out clearly. This is particularly important when prescribing. Examples might include prescribing antibiotics for a respiratory infection, initiating an antihypertensive treatment, or giving an asthmatic a course of steroids. You need to make it explicit to the patient exactly why you are prescribing rather than adopting an expectant approach.

Serious diagnoses

Another problem area is that of the more serious diagnosis that requires a specific action be taken. Candidates seem to assume that you would not be required to actually admit a patient as an emergency or section them in the exam situation, however you should make no assumptions but simply concentrate on making good clinical decisions and taking the appropriate action.

5.13.1 Learning cases

You may find examples of clinical skills assessment cases that have been 'leaked' in some way, either via an Internet forum or from a course. While these can be useful in illustrating the kind of case you will need to deal with, please do be careful. The examiners and administrators are well aware of cases that have reached the public domain and make great efforts to reduce the impact of these leaks. The first step they take is to withdraw the case completely, in which case learning it is not any use to you or your peers at all. The other thing they can do is to change the scenario so it is not immediately recognisable, or actually leave it very similar but change the emphasis or the 'nub' of the case. Writing and rewriting cases is very time consuming and the case-writing examiners' time has to be paid for, so leaking cases actually inflates the cost of what is already a very expensive exam.

Experience in the simulated surgery has shown that candidates who think they know a case tend to do badly! Firstly they make assumptions based on what they have read and these assumptions can be quite misguided especially if the case has been changed. Secondly they often appear to incorporate information they have not visibly gathered, which rather gives the game away to the watching examiner! In this case the examiner will mark accordingly (you are there to demonstrate your technique, not just to come up with the correct diagnosis and treatment). Think of the cases like a maths exam where most of the marks are awarded for the methodology of how you worked the answer out rather than the actual answer itself.

Some experienced examiners hold the view that knowing what cases you are going to see is of very marginal benefit if any at all.

5.14 How to prepare for the exam

We have covered lots of this as we have gone through the various aspects of the consultation, but we will recap in this section.

You have probably picked up by now that passing the clinical skills assessment is about being a good doctor, and in particular being a good consulter. Hopefully you will agree that all the skills we have discussed so far in this chapter are practical, useful skills that make you an effective GP, and that although there are things you can do on the day to improve your chances of passing in general 'examination technique' will count for very little.

Make use of your trainer

Of course there is a bit more to it than simply lots of practice. You need to break down 'being a good doctor' into the specific skills to some extent to focus on each one individually to increase your ability and confidence.

You must also practice integrating these individual skills into your consultations. In chapter 4 we outlined all the various parts of workplace based assessment (the multisource feedback, patient satisfaction questionnaire, consultation observation tool, case based discussion and direct observation of procedural skills). If you thought of these as merely hurdles to get past then you have missed the point — they are there primarily to give you feedback on your performance. Although they are included in your assessment these are primarily formative assessment tools intended to help you understand your strengths and weaknesses and what you need to do to improve. Simply completing the tasks you need to in the workplace based assessment will not get you very far — what you need to do is reflect on each component and consider carefully how to get the most out of it. You can do much of this unassisted, but since the vast majority of it has to be carried out while you are in your time as a GP registrar you have an additional valuable resource, that is your trainer. You really must make sure you get the most you can out of your trainer.

Trainers are experienced GPs with specific training in giving you the individually tailored feedback you need. The nMRCGP might be a new exam but the skills required to pass it are not, and so far as consulting skills are concerned the criteria in the consultation observation tool are very similar to the performance criteria that have been used for some time in the MRCGP video component, so your trainer will be well up to speed on them.

As a GP registrar you have ample opportunity to learn; you get plenty of protected time for learning and specific teaching which for most of you will be one-to-one for much of it. Make sure you put this time to good use. Start video recording yourself early on in your practice attachment and use the recordings as a tool to help you improve. What you will probably find when you watch recordings of yourself consulting is that there are some areas of the consultation you naturally do better in and some you naturally find more difficult. Each week pick an individual area to work on and remind yourself of this at the start of each surgery. When you are focusing on a specific skill, for example exploring the patient's concerns or checking understanding, it is easy enough to reflect at the end of each consultation on how well it went. You do not need to have the video recorder on all the time although when you think you are getting the hang of something it is worth going over some recordings with your trainer to verify that you have indeed improved.

Generally the only time you get to observe a skilled experienced GP consult is in your induction period at the start of your training in general practice. At that stage you are very new to the game and are often concentrating on the bigger picture of the clinical problem and are often relatively oblivious to the subtleties of the consulting skills. You might find it useful to sit in with your trainer and some of the other partners in the practice later on in your time there when you are better able to appreciate what is going on. Try to arrange to sit in on your trainer's surgery when you are preparing for the clinical skills assessment, or persuade your trainer to video record some surgeries. Perhaps the most useful thing to watch for is your trainer's use of time — why is it your trainer can seem to deal with fairly complex problems in less than 10 minutes while you take 15 for simple ones? Is it because experienced doctors cut corners or is it simply that they are more efficient, asking fewer irrelevant questions, being highly selective when it comes to examining a patient, identifying the problem very early on and homing in on it, knowing how to close the consultation efficiently?

Remember that patient-centred consulting is at the heart of the clinical skills assessment. Registrars generally find the listening and explaining skills relatively easier to pick up and put into practice than those required to truly involve the patient in decision-making and in the management plan, so you really need to focus on this. What you should find is that as you get better as it the consultations actually get easier. This should apply to all the consulting skills you are learning but particularly when it comes to formulating a management plan because things are rarely black and white in general practice and there are almost always several different ways of managing a problem, each of which might be equally appropriate. Getting the patient to help you with that process can actually lift the burden and make your life easier.

Consultation models

We have also referred to consultation models. Make sure you understand these and the different features, strengths and weaknesses of each. GP registrars generally think of them as something theoretical that they need to know about because they might get asked about it in an exam. Whilst you certainly might get asked about them in the applied knowledge test, they were developed to help us understand the complex processes going on in the doctor-patient interaction so that we can understand the principles and generalise the learning to apply it elsewhere. Consider which one can help you with each different sort of problem.

Example cases

The College provides some specimen cases on their website and although these are fairly brief they can still be useful. Download them and reflect on the issues raised by each one, how you would attempt to tackle it and what you think the examiners might be looking for. You might be able to persuade your course organiser or programme director to arrange a study day with some role-players and mock cases. If not you can try it within your group without the role-players but doctors do not generally make good role-players so it is far better if you can get some local actors or role-players.

This book now contains an additional chapter containing a selection of cases.

Hopefully the additional detail and guidance in these will be helpful and they can be used as the basis for practice sessions with role-players.

5.14.1 Specific examination techniques

Much of this chapter has, quite rightly, focused on communication skills, but we have also been reminded that your examination technique is important. Make sure you revisit the main bodily systems and remind yourself of a systematic approach to examining the cardiovascular system, respiratory system, the abdomen and the commonly examined parts of the neurological system.

Musculoskeletal complaints are quite easy to reproduce in clinical skills assessment cases, so think of all the various complaints you might meet and remind yourself of the correct technique for examining the back, the shoulder, the hip and knee, etc. Remind yourself of any specific examination techniques that are used, look them up and make them the subject of a tutorial with your trainer. Make sure that as well as learning how to carry out each test you discuss with your trainer the practical merits of each in actually making a diagnosis. Consider even if it would be worth arranging a session in the local orthopaedic clinic to observe some of these being done by the experts? The Arthritis Research Council has prepared a DVD with practical demonstrations of musculoskeletal examinations and although this is aimed at medical students it is a useful resource for preparing for the clinical skills assessment. You can request a free copy from their website.

Here is a quick list of orthopaedic type problems and some of the techniques associated with them:

- Shoulder: can you demonstrate a painful arc correctly and how to test each plane of movement?
- Elbow: think about tennis elbow and golfer's elbow and how you diagnose each
- Wrist: consider carpal tunnel syndrome and tenosynovitis
- Hip: make sure you know how to demonstrate a fixed flexion deformity
- Knee: one of the most complex joints to examine. Can you demonstrate or exclude a joint effusion, test for laxity of the collateral and cruciate ligaments? Are you aware of the specific tests?

All the above are easy enough to revise and become proficient in their performance, that way you can do them fluently in the clinical skills assessment.

5.14.2 Time management

In the MRCGP video you were allowed up to 15 minutes per consultation. This caused examiners some consternation as it did not truly reflect real life since most of us have considerably less time with patients. Also, it led to some very inefficient consulting which was frustrating to watch.

In the clinical skills assessment you will only have 10 minutes with each patient and your preparation must reflect this. When you start your general practice attachment you will of course need longer, but it is important that as you become more proficient you start to work on becoming more efficient and reduce your appointment times. You really should get down to 10 minute appointments at least a month before sitting the assessment. Your trainer and the other partners will be well used to quicker consulting, so it might be worth sitting in a few surgeries with them to see how they keep their consulting times down and make effective use of time.

There are several key skills to time-management within a consultation. One is generally recognising when you have gathered enough information from the patient and shifting the consultation mode slightly into a rather more doctor-centred style. Another is identifying the focus of a consultation quickly and not wasting time down blind alleys. You must also become more proficient at closing consultations.

5.14.3 Courses

Although I will not recommend any specific courses, many registrars will go on a preparatory course for the exam. If you do decide to go on a course, research the courses and see if you can find any feedback from previous candidates. Find out the credentials of the people running the course and doing the teaching — you do not have to be an actual examiner to teach well but of course examiners will have a greater knowledge of the exam and of what you will need to do to pass.

The College hopes to develop a scheme to 'accredit' courses which may help, but remember that just because a course is not accredited it does not mean it is no good. The converse may also be true. You should really look for courses that provide you with an opportunity to practice consultations with role-players, preferably with some expert feedback and guidance.

Attending 'mock' clinical skills assessment sessions, whether organised by your Vocational Training Programme Director or elsewhere, may not be as useful as you expect. Merely practising mock cases is of very limited value alone — after all that is what you are doing in your surgery every day! While it may simulate the pressure of performing in a series of 10 minute consultations what you really need to improve is focused personal feedback.

Similarly do not judge a course or study day based on the number of clinical skills assessment cases you are likely to personally attempt. In reality trainees often learn more from watching their peers consult and the critical factor is receiving expert feedback and teaching from someone who understands exactly what the clinical skills assessment examiners will be looking for and knows exactly how well the key elements of the consultation must be conducted in order to pass. Unfortunately trainees sometimes receive misleading advice from well-meaning tutors who do not actually possess the requisite knowledge of the clinical skills assessment.

Make sure that if you do attend a course you do it early enough to be able to practice anything you learn; you cannot see a complex skill demonstrated one day and perform it yourself the next — it takes time and feedback.

5.15 Attitude

A positive mental attitude is vital. Remember that you have survived medical school, you have got through the selection process to get onto your training scheme, and you have had specific training for the exam. You are reading this book so you know what to expect and how to prepare. You might have been on a course. Visualise the clinical skills assessment as a challenge rather than as a threat — it is a highly valid exam, testing real life skills a GP needs. It is also highly reliable, meaning that if you are good enough you will pass.

Professional athletes and sportsmen understand that mental preparation is key to ensuring they give their best performance on the day of an event. You must do the same for the clinical skills assessment: focus on the things you are doing well in your preparation. When you identify something you can improve see that as a positive, i.e. it is something you can improve rather than the negative aspect of seeing it as something you did badly.

5.16 On the day

5.16.1 Getting there

The clinical skills assessment venue is No 1 Croydon, a purpose-adapted centre in Croydon in the southern suburbs of London. It is well served by public transport, but parking in the area is very limited. Trains run from London Victoria station to East Croydon every few minutes and only take 15 minutes. Make sure you plan your journey well in advance. If you are sitting the assessment in the morning you would be well advised to travel to London and stay overnight the night before. The south east of England is a busy place and transport systems are stretched, as a result any problem tends to result in lots of knock-on delays, so make sure you do not cut it too fine.

Make sure you have a mobile phone with you and the contact number the College have given you. If you are going to be delayed telephone and speak to the administration staff to let them know what has happened and when you think you are likely to arrive. They will do their best to accommodate you or reschedule your exam, but you will appreciate that this may not always be possible. Occasionally candidates or their close relatives get ill or there are significant life events — again telephone the College as soon as you suspect there might be a problem.

The other aspects to getting there relate to what sort of condition you are in when you get there! Make sure you are not getting there sleep-deprived or hung-over. In the final few days before the exam there is little you can do in reality to improve your chances of passing; very little of the assessment is knowledge-based so last minute revision really is not going to help much and can just add to the stress. Plan a relaxing evening before the exam. If you are travelling to London make sure you arrive in plenty of time to unwind and get a good night's sleep. We all have different ways of relaxing whether it be via exercise, reading or socialising therefore choose what works for you. Perhaps think twice about going for that really spicy curry you like unless you are confident you have a cast iron constitution! Most of us perform best if we are well nourished, so make sure you can arrange to have breakfast or lunch before going to the assessment. However do not eat too much as it will make you sleepy.

What you wear is not desperately important; wear what you would normally wear for surgery. It is a professional exam but dressing over formally can affect the consultation so there is no real need for a suit but on the converse turning up in jeans and a T-shirt probably is not going to inspire the patients with much confidence in you.

5.16.2 When you get there

When you get to the exam centre the College's administrative staff will greet and register you. You will need some photographic proof of identity such as photo driving licence or passport. If you do forget it the College staff will do their best to accommodate you to allow you to produce it later, but it is the kind of stress you can do without. You will also be asked to sign a non-disclosure agreement stating that you will not pass on information about the cases to anyone else. The College takes this very seriously and any breaches could be considered a professional issue with significant consequences.

You will be shown into a waiting room with the other candidates — in Croydon there will be three 'circuits' of the exam running at once, each of which will have at least 12 candidates, so there will be up to 40 or so of you. There is a cloakroom and lockers for you to store valuables and any items you are not permitted to take into the exam with you.

Be aware of what suits you best — perhaps you would rather sit quietly or perhaps that just makes you more stressed. You might take some light reading, or engage in conversation (about non-exam related things!) with a fellow-candidate.

For candidates sitting the exam in the afternoon there's a 'quarantine' period during which you are not allowed to leave the waiting room. This is to prevent you from meeting candidates leaving the morning sitting and potentially discussing the cases with them.

There will be a briefing before you are shown to your consulting room. This will be delivered by one of the senior examiners and as well as clarifying what you should expect it will remind you of the exam regulations. These will be rigorously enforced and anyone found cheating risks disqualification. You will be given the opportunity to ask questions at the end of the briefing, following which a marshal will lead you to your room. The marshals are also senior examiners so will be able to answer questions for you if need be.

Once in your consulting room you will have a little time to settle down and get your equipment ready. You can also read the briefing instructions on your desk and have a look at the patient notes — they will be arranged in the order in which you will see the patients. Do you benefit from looking through the whole list? You have probably noticed for yourself that knowing who is coming to see you in a surgery can be off-putting if you notice a couple of heartsink patients in the list, and the same applies here. There is a strong case to be made to read the notes for the first patient and leave it at that. There will not be much in the patient notes: you will be given their name, age and sex, any significant past history and any recent history of note or relevant investigation results or hospital letters and/or investigations.

You are allowed to write on the patient's notes and this is purely for your own benefit and will not be seen by the examiner. You might wish to write a couple of prompts: these could be generic, for example reminding yourself to smile and use open questions, or case specific, such as a reminder about specific questions or information form the *British National Formulary* on a specific drug.

5.16.3 Equipment
You are allowed to take a normal doctor's bag with its usual contents into the exam with you. This includes a stethoscope, otoscope, ophthalmoscope, etc. You are also allowed to take in a *British National Formulary* and *Children's British National Formulary*. You will have been sent a comprehensive list of what is allowed and what is not when you apply for the exam, and you will be reminded again in the briefing. Generally speaking you are not allowed any other books, protocols or guidelines, and you are not allowed any electronic equipment, including mobile phones. You are not allowed to take a desktop clock into your room with you to help you keep track of time mainly because some candidates were using digital timers with for example a warning 'bleep' at nine minutes, which was distracting to the role-player. Each consulting room has a large clock on the wall quite low down and immediately in front of you so it is easy to see without turning away from the patient.

If you get there and find you have forgotten something, do not panic! If it comes to a physical examination, role-play it and explain that you have forgotten your equipment. It is unlikely to influence your marks.

You are allowed to take a drink and snack into your room if you wish and water fountains and plastic cups are provided on each examining floor.

5.16.4 Behaving naturally
The key to performing on the day is to simply be a good doctor. Concentrate on the skills we have discussed in this chapter and try to be as relaxed and natural

as you can. Concentrate entirely on the patient and ignore the examiner, who will do their best to be unobtrusive and keep out of your line of sight. Do not look to the examiner for cues — imagine it is just you and the patient in the room.

You will naturally feel nervous, possibly very nervous, but remind yourself that it is to be expected and that everyone else is in the same boat! Remember also that a degree of stress heightens alertness and can improve performance, so do not perceive your nervousness as a negative. It will usually settle within seconds of the first patient coming into your room in any case.

Be nice to the patient, decide how to introduce yourself and smile — it will make you and the patient feel better.

You will be really surprised how natural it can feel. The role-players are very good, the cases are realistic and well written and you will feel like you are in a real consultation. Do not try to second guess what the examiners want from you, just concentrate on doing your best for the patient in front of you. There are no tricks or traps, and any hidden agendas will be realistic and if you give them a chance the role-players will give you ample opportunity to spot them.

Do not try to think what the College 'party line' is on issues, just concentrate on good medical practice as appropriate for a normal GP.

5.16.5 The actual surgery

At the start of the surgery there will be a buzzer and your first patient will knock and walk in. While you are greeting the patient the examiner will come in behind them and take a seat towards the back of the room. They should be positioned so that they are not in either your or the patient's immediate line of sight. They are briefed not to greet you or make eye contact, so do not feel offended and do not try to engage with them.

You can write on the paperwork provided, but be aware that it can be distracting for the patient as well as for yourself. You do not need to keep any record of the consultation and anything you write will not be seen by the examiner or contribute to your marks in any way. You have no computer to worry about and no risk of telephone interruptions so you have no excuses for giving the patient anything less than 100% of your attention.

You will have 13 consultations in total, of which 12 will be marked and the other will be a case that is being piloted. You will not know which one that is, so do not worry about it and consider them all equally important. It is possible that you will have a video camera in your room, if so it will be an unobtrusive closed circuit television camera rather than a stand alone camera on a tripod and you are unlikely to notice it. The purpose of this is for quality control and training purposes, to allow the examiners to check that a case is working as planned, to monitor the role-players' performances and the calibration of the examiners. It is not there to record your performance.

After the 10 minutes is up there will be another buzzer to mark the end of the consultation. You need to close the consultation quickly — it is no good keeping on talking trying to get a few last points in because if you do that the role-player will simply get up and leave, and in any case the examiner is not likely to give you any credit for a few quick garbled instructions. It is best to simply say goodbye.

Remember to relax between patients and focus on the next patient you are going to see rather than dwell on the last one – remember Roger Neighbour's 'housekeeping' points. Thoughts on the consultation you have just done will inevitably tend to be negative, so instead think about how you are going to approach the next patient, or even think about something completely unrelated such as what you are going to do when you get home. You will have a couple of minutes break before the next patient comes in as it takes a little time for the examiner to complete the mark sheet and move on to the next consulting room with the role-player. Occasionally it may take a little longer, perhaps because there are problems with paperwork or a role-player or the examiner might need to be swapped around. Do not worry, just stay in your room and wait. Familiarise yourself with the notes for the next patient and write down any prompts you think might be useful on their notes.

After the seventh case there will be a refreshment break. Wait in your room until a marshal collects you to take you to the refreshment area for tea/coffee and biscuits. There are also toilet facilities in this area. The break will last between 20 and 30 minutes, during which time you may chat with your fellow candidates, however an invigilator will be present to make sure you do not discuss the cases. You will not be allowed to use your mobile phone during the break.

At the end of the surgery you should wait in your room until a marshal tells you may leave. Make sure you gather all your bits of equipment and collect your belongings from your locker. You must not remove any of the paperwork from your desk, and this includes any rough notes you have made — the College takes the security of the case bank very seriously.

5.16.6 Concerns

Rarely things happen that you feel might have compromised your ability to perform well in the exam. This could be something to do with the role-player's behaviour or performance, the examiner's behaviour or something entirely extraneous. While the role-players and examiners are highly professional, they are also human, so you do need to be realistic about this. If the role-player does make a slip or perform sub-optimally the examiner will almost certainly notice this before you do and will compensate for this in the grading. Similarly role-players and examiners get minor illnesses like colds and hayfever and you may need to accept a bit of sniffing or sneezing for example.

Each examiner has a clipboard with lots of pieces of paperwork including the role-player briefing, the marking schedule, your personalised mark sheet and there may well be a little shuffling of paperwork going on. Again the examiner will try to do this as quietly as possible.

If you do feel something has affected your performance, however, it is best to ask to speak to the marshal — there will be a senior marshal on each circuit of the exam and they will listen to and note your concerns. It is best to do this either during the break in the middle of the surgery or at the end. They will do their best to rectify any problems at the time, but if that is not possible they will document it and take it up and correspond with you later. The MRCGP exam has always had an impeccable reputation for fairness and all those involved want it to remain that way.

5.17 After the exam

It could well be that the clinical skills assessment is the last part of your exam. In any case it will still be an anti-climax after all the preparation. A long train journey home alone can be a bit miserable after a stressful experience, so investigate if you have the opportunity to meet up with friends or have your partner meet you for an evening out in London. If you have friends sitting the assessment at the same time as you then you will inevitably have a debrief, but again it is best not to dwell on your perceived mistakes and missed opportunities. The problem with debriefs is that they rarely make you feel any better about an exam! You never focus on the cases you did well, instead remembering only the ones you struggled with where you think you made a mistake.

It is inevitable that you will discuss the cases you have encountered with your colleagues back in your practice and on your training scheme, but there is a difference between having a chat about the cases and actually trying to create a written record of them. In addition to the non-disclosure agreement you have signed, it is unprofessional to attempt to compromise the exam. The reason the College wants to maintain the confidentiality of the case bank is to maintain the fairness of the exam. Another point is that the cases in the clinical skills assessment case bank number in the hundreds and are rotated regularly so your friends are unlikely to see the same cases anyway and could waste their time and effort on working up cases they will never see. As I pointed out previously, there is even a risk that knowing a case might compromise a candidate's performance rather than improving it.

Hopefully you will be able to celebrate when the results come out. It is a very rewarding feeling when you pass a challenging exam, and although the clinical skills assessment is challenging, hopefully you will regard it as having been a fair and valid assessment of your abilities as a GP. Of course passing the nMRCGP is actually a starting point not only for your career in general practice but also for your membership of the Royal College of General Practitioners. The RCGP is unique amongst the medical Royal Colleges in having a highly devolved organisation with local Faculties. Why not get involved with your local Faculty? Most Faculty Boards are only too delighted to see enthusiastic young GPs getting involved.

Finally, good luck!

Balint M (2000) *The Doctor, his Patient and the Illness*. 2nd edn. Churchill Livingstone, London

Byrne PS, Long BEL (1976) *Doctors Talking to Patients*. Royal College of General Practitioners, London

Edwards A, Elwyn G, Mulley A (2002) Explaining risks: turning numerical data into meaningful pictures. *BMJ* **324**: 827–30

Elyn G, Edwards A, Gwyn R et al (1999) Towards a feasible model for shared decision-making: focus group study with general practice registrars. *BMJ* **319**: 753–56

Neighbour R, et al (2004) *The Inner Consultation: How to Develop an Effective and Intuitive Consulting Style*. Radcliffe Publishing, Oxford

Pendleton D, Schofield T Tate P, Havelock P (1984) *The Consultation — An Approach to Teaching and Learning*. Oxford University Press, Oxford

Stott NC, Davis RH (1979) The exceptional potential in each primary care consultation. *J R Coll Gen Pract* **29**: 201-5

Tate P (2006) *The Doctor's Communication Handbook*. Radcliffe Publishing, Oxford

Resources

Breaking Bad News: *www.breakingbadnews.co.uk*

General Medical Council: *www.gmc-uk.org*

Royal College of General Practitioners: *www.rcgp.org.uk*

Arthritis Research Council: *www.arc.org.uk*

CHAPTER 6

Examples of clinical skills assessment cases

This chapter contains some sample clinical skills assessment cases. These cases have all been written by myself for teaching purposes on the Swansea MRCGP course. Any similarity to any other cases, either genuine nMRCGP cases or otherwise is purely coincidental and reflects the fact that there is in fact a limited number of 'themes' on which to base cases.

The format of the cases is similar, but not identical, to that of genuine clinical skills assessment cases. I have included fairly full role-player briefings mainly to give you some idea of the amount and nature of the information given to role-players to enable them to enact the cases consistently and reliably. It will also allow you to use these cases with role-players for teaching and practice purposes, but once you have read the role-player briefings and discussion you will probably get little benefit from actually trying them out since the briefings generally give the game away. I have not included formal marking schedules but for each case have given clear indications as to what an examiner would be looking for in terms of having both a positive as well as negative effect on grading. I have also included potential pitfalls. For most of the cases much of the consulting behaviour required is given away in the role-player briefing.

List of cases

1. An abnormal scan
2. A raised PSA
3. Memory loss
4. Tired all the time
5. Leg pain
6. A request to change treatment ~ read
7. Complaint
8. Acne ~ read
9. Back pain
10. Foot pain
11. Deafness
12. Pre-menstrual syndrome
13. Convulsion
14. Depression

1. An abnormal scan

Overview
A female patient attends for the result of an ultrasound scan. The scan suggests the possibility of a carcinoma.

What the case is designed to test
The candidate's ability to break bad news and offer ongoing support.

Role-player briefing
You are Clare B, a 35-year-old single woman. About a month ago you found a small lump in your neck. You came to the doctor to get it checked out. The doctor you saw thought it was your thyroid gland and arranged an ultrasound scan and a blood test. You have come back today for the results. The doctor you saw, Dr. Morgan, was generally pretty reassuring — he thought it might be a cyst — and you were not particularly worried.

You work as a primary school teacher and live alone. You do not have a boyfriend at the moment. Your parents are both alive but live 50 miles away. You are generally fit and well with no past medical history and you are not taking any treatment.

You had not experienced any other symptoms — the lump is not painful or tender and you are generally well. You have not lost any weight.

Opening statement
'I've come back for my results doctor.'

How to behave
You need to be surprised when the doctor tells you he/she has bad news, you thought it was going to be OK and really did not expect to be told you might have a cancer. Try to display a degree of denial by saying: *'But Dr. Morgan said he thought it was just a cyst'*, or *'But it can't be a cancer, I feel so well'*, etc. Try not to overplay it, no histrionics and try to avoid actually crying. Do not say too much, sit fairly quietly and let the doctor do most of the talking.

If the doctor uses vague terms like 'growth', 'mass', 'abnormality', etc. you need to ask what he/she means; you are not sure if they mean it is a cancer or not unless they actually use the word 'cancer'.

Once the doctor has explained the result you want to know what will happen next. It is likely the doctor will volunteer most of this but if not you need to ask about how quickly you will be seen by the specialist, if you might need any other tests, what treatment you might have and of course how serious it is. Although you are fairly well educated you do not have a medical background and you know very little about cancer and have never heard of cancer of the thyroid.

If the doctor asks if there is anyone who can come to be with you or collect you say there is not really but that you will be OK, and that you will probably ring your mum when you get home. If the doctor suggests it might be a good idea to come back in a day or two when it has sunk in a bit be prepared to accept the offer.

Dress casually. Try not to be over-emotional and try to avoid displaying any anger even if you feel the doctor is not doing very well or is irritating you. This is quite a challenging case anyway and having too much emotion can make it too challenging. Try not to help the doctor too much but bear the following:

* If they spend too long on the preamble before giving you the diagnosis give them some cues, either verbal or non-verbal, that you are a bit impatient to get the actual result
* Deciding exactly when to introduce the concept of 'cancer' is sometimes quite difficult for the doctor, if they use vague terms that do not make it clear that it is cancer or if they seem to be presenting a fairly optimistic outlook it can be helpful to collude with them by saying *'so it is not cancer then doctor?'*, which should push them in the right direction.

Patient notes
* Clare B, age 35.
* Last seen four weeks ago (by Dr Morgan)
* Noticed lump in left side of neck. On examination 1cm diameter lump appears to be in thyroid, ?cyst.
* For ultrasound scan and TFT.
* 1 week ago: TFT: TSH 2.4, T4 18 (normal)
* Ultrasound: there is a 1cm solid mass within the left lobe of the thyroid gland. Scan otherwise normal. Malignancy is highly probable and an urgent surgical opinion is suggested.

Discussion
This is quite a challenging case as breaking bad news to a patient is difficult, especially if, as in this case, the patient is not expecting it. It should however be immediately obvious to the candidate where the focus of the case lies and in fact this is a case where having sight of the patient notes before you see the patient does tell you pretty much exactly what the case is going to be about. This allows you to plan your approach: remind yourself that establishing rapport with this patient is vitally important, although it would be inappropriate to be too cheerful! Remind yourself of the principles you have been taught previously about breaking bad news.

The role-player briefing does of course contain lots of hints about what you should and should not be doing in this case! The good candidate will establish rapport quickly and will take a minute or so establishing the background by asking something like: '*Would you mind just running over what's led to you having the scan and what happened when you saw Dr Morgan?*'. You should also ask if Dr Morgan gave any indication as to what he expected to find, and explore whether the patient herself had any particular worries. However beware wasting too much time with the preamble — it should be immediately obvious to you that you have quite a lot of ground to cover in breaking the news and discussing future management with the patient.

It probably would not be good to read out the ultrasound report verbatim since it gives the diagnosis away quite starkly. You need to introduce the bad news gently by saying something like: '*I'm afraid the scan shows an abnormality*', or: '*I'm afraid it shows a lump in your thyroid gland*', and wait for a response from the patient. If the patient takes the hint and asks if it is serious then you should then take the opportunity to confirm that it is and give an honest explanation. If the patient however appears to assume this still is not terribly serious you need to act quite quickly but sensitively to correct this. You need to introduce the suggestion that the lump is probably cancerous quite early on.

The patient at this stage is going to be upset, so you must demonstrate empathy. Do what you would normally do in surgery; some of us are more tactile than others and using touch clumsily can be counter-productive. Take your time, and allow the patient to gather her thoughts and ask questions.

You need to explain the diagnosis. Thyroid cancer is relatively rare so you probably know very little, if anything, about the prognosis, what treatment is required, etc. and it has been deliberately chosen for this case for those reasons. If you do happen to know lots about thyroid cancer then fine, but for most of us it is best to offer generic advice and leave the details to the specialist you are going to refer her to. The patient is likely to have lots of questions that you cannot answer and therefore it is best to be honest and say that you cannot answer them rather than speculating and potentially misleading the patient. You need to formulate a management plan and while you do not know what treatment she is going to require, you do know lots of things:

- The two-week rule applies so you can promise an early appointment with the specialist
- It is going to require further investigation, possibly a biopsy
- She is going to needs lots of support in the near future
- It will help enormously if you make it clear that you are taking the problem seriously and will take personal responsibility for ensuring you will be there for her, to answer questions, coordinate her care, etc.
- You cannot possibly expect to answer all her questions in this single consultation.

While being open about the diagnosis you should provide positive reassurance that you will do your best for her. Allow her to ask questions. Be very positive about what is going to happen next with time scales. This is a life changing event for this patient so it is not unreasonable to 'pull out all the stops' and personally contact the local hospital to talk about an appointment.

Perhaps she'd like you to contact someone to come and collect her — is she in any fit state to drive herself home? Perhaps offer to let her sit quietly in another room, and/or perhaps offer to spend more time with her at the end of surgery. You should certainly arrange further contact with her in the near future.

There is lots to think of and lots to do, and unless you are a superhuman you will not fit it all in, so do not worry unduly if you run out of time.

Marking domains

This case is clearly predominantly in the domain of interpersonal skills. You are given the diagnosis so information gathering does not really come into it, but the clinical management domain is relevant.

The examiner will be looking for you establishing rapport, breaking the news with empathy but without ambiguity, formulating a sensible management plan and making sure the patient is clear about this.

Pitfalls for this case including appearing cold, too blunt, taking too long breaking the news, being ambiguous about it being a cancer (i.e. colluding with a patient in denial), and not managing the patient appropriately once the news has been broken.

This is potentially quite an emotional case so once consultation has ended you will need to gather yourself together and focus on the next case. No matter how well you have performed it is unlikely you will feel you have done well here!

2. Raised PSA

Overview
A middle aged man presents with a borderline PSA.

What the case is designed to test
- The candidate's ability to explain the meaning of a borderline abnormal result and its implications for the patient
- Ability to help the patient make an informed choice regarding further action.

Role-player briefing
You are David J, a 55-year-old (age not really terribly important) accountant and for about six months have noticed that you need to get up in the night to pass urine — lately it has been three or four times a night. You also notice that the stream is not as good as it used to be and it takes longer to empty your bladder. About two weeks ago you saw your usual doctor (Dr Smith) who performed a rectal examination and told you that your prostate gland was slightly enlarged. He also arranged for you to have a blood test three days later (it is fairly important that it was three days later) and you have come back today for the result.

You have had no other symptoms — no trouble starting or stopping passing urine, no blood in the urine and you are otherwise fit and well. If the doctor asks about any other symptoms reply in the negative.

You have heard that the prostate gland enlarges as men get older and suspect that this is what's been happening to you. You had not really been worried about cancer until Dr Smith mentioned the possibility. You do not know much about the blood test except that it is a test for prostate cancer. Since seeing Dr Smith you have been a little bit worried about it but not terribly and you expect it will probably be normal. While you are naturally concerned when the doctor mentions cancer it is important not to over-react to this — if you become terribly worried about it this will result in the doctor feeling the only option is to refer you for further investigations and the point of this case is to explore the doctor's ability to explain the pros and cons of further investigation and help you to make an informed choice.

Opening statement
'I've come back for my blood test result doctor.'

How to behave
You should wear a suit or smart casual clothing, as befits an accountant.

You are an intelligent man and while you are neither particularly deferential towards the doctor or 'pushy' you would appreciate a full explanation and to have some say in what happens.

If the doctor says the test result is abnormal you should ask if this means you have cancer. If the doctor plays down the abnormality you should say: *'So I don't have cancer then?'*.

The doctor might try to find out more about what you know about the test before telling you — if so be fairly neutral, say you have only heard of the test and know only that it is a test for prostate cancer but not much else. If asked if you have any worries about it say that you were not really worried and that you expected the test would probably be normal.

If the doctor expresses the result in numbers, for example telling you it is 8, ask what that means. If he expresses it in terms of abnormality by saying it is either abnormal or borderline, ask how abnormal it is. Try to get the doctor to explain what the numbers mean and try to get him to quantify the risk of you having cancer. You as an accountant and are used to working with numbers and think it is not too much to expect for the doctor to give you a 'yes' or 'no' answer. If the doctor uses terms like 'suspicious' or 'malignancy' ask if he means cancer. You need to show an appropriate level of concern at the mention of prostate cancer, also if the doctor starts talking about what sounds quite unpleasant investigations or treatment, but do not overdo this.

If the doctor suggests that you should be referred for further investigations ask exactly what investigations he thinks you need and how important it is that you have them. You do not like hospitals much and are not keen on having any painful or unpleasant investigations unless the doctor can reassure you of the benefit, but do not volunteer this information unless the doctor asks. Do not let the doctor get away with using medical jargon and ask him (politely, without irritation) to explain any medical terms he uses such as 'biopsy'. If the doctor seems to be making a clear decision to refer you to a specialist you should ask lots of questions about what is going to happen to you and indicate non-verbally that you do not like the sound of it.

Ask the doctor about what treatment might be offered and ask all the obvious questions about how unpleasant it is, how successful it is, what the side effects are, etc. Also ask what might happen if you did not have investigations and treatment.

If however the doctor suggests waiting and repeating the test you should express a little more concern about the suspicion of a cancer and ask about any risks in delaying further investigation. If the doctor gives an explanation and wants to know what you would prefer to do, you find this a difficult decision to make. It might be appropriate to ask the doctor what he/she would do in your situation.

Patient notes
- David J, age 55.
- No past medical history of note
- Last seen two weeks ago (by Dr Smith, practice partner)
- Nocturia x 3-4, poor stream, several months
- No other symptoms
- PR: smooth moderately enlarged prostate

- Clinically BPH. Check PSA in few days and review
- 1 week ago: Serum PSA 4.5ug/l (normal up to 3.5ug/l)

Discussion

Again the role-player briefing pretty much gives away the nub of the case — dealing with the uncertainty surrounding a borderline result. Using PSA to test for prostate malignancy is topical and an issue you will almost certainly have encountered before. You do not require much in the way of factual knowledge to tackle the case other than what investigations would be likely in the event of a referral and what treatment the patient might be offered.

Dealing with a borderline PSA can be tricky since it is not a terribly sensitive or specific test. Also there is not a definitive treatment suitable for early disease since most options have fairly horrendous side-effects (impotence, incontinence, etc.) and there is little evidence that early intervention improves mortality. The next stage in investigating is probably a transrectal biopsy of the prostate which is not terribly pleasant. Basically there is not a clear cut correct answer as to whether this patient should be referred or not.

The answer of course lies in exploring this patient's personal preferences and values. Considerable skill is required in explaining the implications of the test and any further investigations/treatment, and the good candidate will guide the patient towards a decision.

Marking domains

This is probably fairly evenly balanced between clinical management and interpersonal skills with minimal information-gathering.

Clearly the examiner will not be impressed with a doctor-centred approach or with a poor explanation. However be wary of the opposite extreme, that of abdicating the responsibility to the patient and leaving him to make a decision alone. If the patient asks you what you think he should do give your honest opinion and justify it to him. This applies whether you feel he should be investigated right away or whether you feel a more expectant approach is reasonable.

Whether you actually refer or not is largely irrelevant so far as passing the case is concerned, it is all about the process. Interestingly when I have used this case in groups of trainees many have leaned heavily towards referring but when asked what they would want for themselves would prefer to monitor the situation!

3. Memory loss

Overview
A daughter attends expressing concern about her father's memory. She does not want him to know she has come to see you.

What the case is designed to test
- Being able to conduct a third party consultation appropriately
- Make a risk assessment
- Formulate/negotiate a pragmatic solution to the problem including involving other agencies such as social services and a psychogeriatrician.

Role-player briefing
You are Clare L and you have booked an appointment to see the doctor to discuss your father (Edward L, age 67) with his doctor. For some time you and your brother have been aware that your father is becoming increasingly forgetful. Initially you poked fun at him but lately you have become worried that he might be developing Alzheimer's disease.

What has triggered the consultation is that last week you called in to see him and found a pan boiled dry still on a hot stove. Your dad was in the living room watching TV and had clearly forgotten about it. He was fairly dismissive of it and said it was a simple slip anyone could make. He also occasionally seems to forget which day it is — he was surprised one Saturday when you called round as he thought it was a weekday and expected you to be in work. Ha also seems to have got into the habit of writing things down on bits of paper to remind himself of things he needs to do like putting the bins out and doing the shopping. You suspect he sometimes eats twice because he has forgotten that he has already eaten (you found two sets of dirty dishes in the kitchen one afternoon). When you have tried to talk to him about it he gets a bit angry and says there is nothing wrong with him. You did suggest he come to see the doctor but he said there was no need and refused. You suspect he will be quite angry if he knows you have been to see the doctor about him without him knowing.

You have talked to your brother about it and he agrees with you that it is a problem and wonders whether your dad should go into a home.

You have heard of Alzheimer's disease and know that it causes memory loss and confusion. You are worried that he might be unsafe living alone and wonder what might be done to help. You are sure he would not agree to going into a home and wonder if there is any way he could have some supervision at home. You also saw a TV programme about Alzheimer's disease that talked about drug treatment but said that it was difficult to get it on the NHS.

Your goals for this consultation are to see if the doctor agrees about the problem and to see what he/she suggests.

Your dad is a retired policeman and has been fit all his life. Your mum died of a heart attack five years ago. Your dad does not smoke but goes down to the local pub with his friends a couple of times a week. He is not a heavy drinker. Both you and your brother work full time. You are a secretary, your brother is a bus driver and you both have families. There is no way either of you could do much more than you are doing already — between the two of making sure one of you calls in each day to check he is OK and you take it in turns to have him over to your own house on a Sunday.

Your Dad lives in a semi-detached house with gas central heating and an electric cooker. He does have a gas fire in his living room that he often puts on in the evening. His neighbours are friendly but are all out working during the week.

Opening statement
'I've come because I'm worried about my father's memory, he's been getting quite forgetful recently.'

How to behave
Try not to give too much information away initially, just tell the doctor about the pan incident and wait for him/her to ask you more questions. Wait till the doctor asks before you admit that your dad does not know you have come to see the doctor. Do not mention your brother unless the doctor asks about family or if you have discussed the problem with anyone else, or if it seems likely the doctor will end the consultation without asking. Do not mention the TV programme unless the doctor asks you what you know about Alzheimer's disease.

If the doctor asks how you thought he/she might be able to help just say that you wanted to see what he/he thought could be done. Stress that you do not want him to know that you have come — the doctor is unlikely to be happy to collude with this idea and if he/she comes up with what you feel are plausible arguments you will go along with whatever the doctor suggests. If the doctor more or less refuses to do anything because your dad has not approached him/her of his own free will you need to put a bit of pressure on for something to be done but without becoming angry.

The doctor is likely to want to do some or all of the following:

- Make an assessment of your dad's mental state him/herself
- Arrange an assessment by a psychiatrist for the elderly
- Arrange an assessment by the practice's health visitor (in which case ask what the health visitor does)
- Arrange to contact social services for an assessment.

Make sure you are perfectly clear about exactly what the doctor plans to do and when. Is there anything you can do in the meantime to help?

If the doctor suggests a 'wait and see' approach you will be very unhappy to accept this and will ask if that means waiting till your dad burns the house down or something.

Patient notes
- Edward L, age 67
- 15 years ago — inguinal hernia repair
- 10 years ago — reflux symptoms, prescribed antacid
- October last year — flu vaccine clinic. Vaccine given, BP 132/85

Discussion
This case would be much more straightforward if it were not for the fact that the daughter does not want her father to know she has come to you. While her position is understandable it is fairly unrealistic!

Clearly you are going to want to make an assessment of Mr. Lewis' mental state but there is sufficient in the history to make it clear he almost certainly has dementia and is at some degree of risk. Doing nothing is therefore clearly not an option and you will need to think creatively how you manage this. There are several options including:

- Talk her round into allowing you to explain to him why you are seeing him and arrange to visit
- Arrange to visit and assess anyway with some other excuse for the visit
- Consider something more creative like inviting him in for a routine health check

You should certainly attempt to persuade her that it is going to be difficult to do anything without engaging with him. Perhaps she is right that he may be angry, but you can explain that she is acting in his best interests, etc. The ideal situation would be that she persuade him to come to see you (hopefully accompanied by her), or agree for you to visit him.

Mr. Lewis' *autonomy* is an important issue here; he clearly has the right not to see a doctor and not to have his mental health assessed. However since there is enough evidence for you to believe he is at some risk, which is only likely to get worse, it is reasonable to take the view that it is in his best interests that you get involved. Forcing any management options on him is another issue entirely though!

Beware of using the fact that he does not know she is here as grounds to refuse to get involved — if you feel he is at risk you have a responsibility towards him. You should empathise with the daughter and make it clear that you agree that you should become involved and that you are taking her concerns seriously. There is also a lot of guilt here so you should do what you can to alleviate this by reassuring her that she has done the right thing in coming to you and that you will do what you can to persuade her father to see it this way.

The daughter wants you to come up with some practical suggestions and it is reasonable to discuss the possibilities with her on the assumption that your subsequent assessment confirms the dementia. You need to think of practical options that can be offered; these are likely to include involving the local psychogeriatrician and his team including the community psychogeriatric nurse, and possibly social services. You have hopefully already identified two specific risks — the electric hob and the gas fire. A microwave oven is a much safer way of heating food and perhaps there are alternatives to the open gas fire.

Marking domains

This case is perhaps fairly evenly split between all three domains — you are going to need good information gathering skills, some creative management planning and the interpersonal skills to empathise with the daughter and try to talk her round.

As in most cases there are no set pass/fail criteria. As in all clinical skills assessment cases, concentrate on identifying the problem then in addressing it. If the examiner feels that the daughter is leaving the room feeling that it was worth coming to see you and that something meaningful is going to come of it you have probably passed as long as your suggestions are medically plausible and acceptable.

4. Tired all the time

Overview
A patient complaining of being tired all the time with no evidence of physical or psychiatric morbidity.

What the case is designed to test
The ability to take a detailed history to exclude any significant physical or psychiatric illness, provide an adequate explanation and negotiate an appropriate management plan.

Role-player briefing
You are Chloe R, a 28-year-old single schoolteacher. For the last three months or so you have just been feeling tired all the time. You have no energy, when you get home from school in the evening you do not feel like doing anything and often fall asleep while watching the TV. You often go to bed early, before 9pm, and you struggle to wake up when the alarm goes off at 7.30am, feeling like you have not slept at all. At weekends you stay asleep often till lunchtime.

Your relationship with your boyfriend is fine although lately you have seen a bit less of him because you are just too tired to go out in the evenings. You have been teaching in a local junior school for the last five years and there are no problems there, you get on fine with your work colleagues. You used to go to the gym regularly and run occasionally but you have not had the energy recently — it is all you can do to muster up the energy to take your dog out for a walk at the weekends.

You are generally fit and healthy, your appetite seems OK, and your weight has not changed. You do not feel depressed although you are getting fed up of being tired all the time and are worried there is something wrong with you. You do still enjoy socialising and watching TV, etc. but just feel tired all the time. You have tried eating a healthy diet but it does not seem to have made a difference. You do not smoke and drink a few glasses of wine at weekends. If the doctor asks about any other specific symptoms answer in the negative. Your periods are regular and you are on the contraceptive pill.

Opening statement
'I'm feeling tired all the time doctor.'

How to behave
If the doctor asks open questions explain about the sleeping all the time, the lack of energy, etc. Be prepared to freely volunteer all the information in the first paragraph above but only give the rest in response to specific questions.

It is fairly important you do not give the impression that you are depressed and if the doctor presses this line of questioning you should state that you really do not feel depressed with appropriate body language to convince them.

If asked what you think the cause is say that you have no idea, but that you have been worried there must be something causing it. If the doctor asks about myalgic encelophalopathy (ME) say that you have heard of it but had not really considered it. You have not heard of chronic fatigue syndrome.

If the doctor asks to examine you ask what they want to look for. If they press, decline a physical examination — the examiner will tell them everything is normal.

It is quite likely the doctor will suggest some blood tests — ask which ones and whether they think they will give them the answer. Ask what happens next if they come back as normal.

Be prepared to accept whatever explanations the doctor offers but ask what can be done about it.

Patient notes
* Chloe R, age 28
* No past medical history of note.

Discussion
Here is a classic general practice problem, an otherwise apparently healthy patient who complains of feeling tired all the time. It is such a common problem that we all recognise the abbreviation to 'TATT'. It can be a heartsink problem as we often do not uncover a cause and we often cannot come up with a solution.

The key here is to be patient-centred and elicit everything you can from the patient, then conduct a methodical enquiry to exclude the more significant medical problems. It is important that you conduct the consultation with a fairly open mind. The lack of other physical symptoms (the lack of weight loss should be reassuring) means that an underlying physical illness is unlikely although it is wise to check a full blood count and thyroid function test to exclude anaemia and hypothyroidism. Dr. Bill Jerrett, a GP in South Wales, published a case series in the early 80s clearly demonstrating a low return rate from these investigations, however it is wise to carry them out. It was pointed out in chapter 5 that negative investigations do not always reassure patients. What some of the research does suggest is that communication skills are key and that if the patient knows exactly what you are trying to exclude in the test then that can be helpful, therefore perhaps explain that occasionally patients with tiredness can be anaemic or have an underactive thyroid and that you want to make sure it is not either of those.

You should also question carefully to exclude depression — as you can see from the briefing the role-player is carefully briefed not to send you down this path and in the actual clinical skills assessment the examiners and role-players will spend a lot of time on this to make sure it is got right.

Marking domains
The emphasis is slightly weighted towards the information gathering domain

here since a careful history and targeted mental state examination to exclude depression are important. Your clinical management and interpersonal skills are still required however.

The biggest risk here is of the candidate deciding early on that this is a depressed patient. It is fine to generate this as a hypothesis early on, but you must put in the due diligence to check this out carefully.

The examiner will not be looking for any specific management plan but will be looking to see if you have addressed the patient's problem and made her feel it was worthwhile coming to see you. Think about how you would explain tiredness to your patients.

5. Leg pain

Overview
A teenager presents with pain in his lower leg for two months.

What the case is designed to test
- Taking a history and performing an examination
- Correctly identify a potentially serious problem
- Explain the differential diagnosis without being either unduly reassuring or alarming.

Role-player briefing
You are Chris S, a 16-year-old who has just started A-levels and for a couple of months now you have been having an aching pain in your right leg. It is below the knee and although it is not terribly severe it seems to have slowly got worse. It does not bother you when you walk, cycle or play football but it sometimes aches a little bit more afterwards. You are aware of it in the night and it has been bad enough to wake you sometimes during the last couple of weeks.

You are generally fit and healthy and have never had any serious illnesses. You have taken an ibuprofen occasionally which seems to relieve the pain for a while. You are eating OK and have had a bit of a growth spurt recently.

Your mum reckons it is what she calls 'growing pains' but when you asked her what that meant she did not really seem to be able to explain it for you. You looked it up on the Internet and that was not much help either and you were not sure that fitted your problem and seems to affect younger children than yourself. You really have no ideas about it but think it is probably something minor and have only come because your mum said you should. She did not come with you today because she is at work (works in a shop).

Opening statement
'My mum thinks I'm having growing pains doctor.'

How to behave
You need to try not to volunteer too much information initially, let the doctor ask you some questions. Try to decide how much to give away and when based on how the doctor makes you feel, but do not be obstructive. You need to try to appear relaxed — you are not too worried about this pain. It is fairly important that the pain is not worse when you exercise, and that it is only slightly worse after exercise. Do not immediately volunteer that it has been waking you at night.

You should try to find out what the doctor thinks it might be. If the doctor wants to arrange any tests (blood tests, X-rays, etc.) you should ask if he/she thinks it might be serious. If they say they do you need to try to get them to explain more — you have not for a minute thought it might be anything serious and will be suitably worried.

If the doctor says he/she wants to see you with your mum or dad say you can arrange that but you should still try to find out as much as you can for yourself first. If the doctor asks about family history say your granddad has some arthritis in his knees but you do not know of anything else. Answer 'no' to any other symptoms the doctor might ask you.

Wear normal teenager attire but ideally shorts so that the doctor can examine your leg.

There are no abnormal findings, the leg is not tender anywhere. If the doctor asks you to point to where the pain is point to the shin bone about 10cm below the knobbly bit just below the knee. Check this with the examiner before playing the role.

You should pitch your attitude somewhere between being a sullen monosyllabic teenager and a confident, articulate one. Do not make life too difficult for the doctor but do not be too forthcoming. Try to adjust your behaviour depending on how well you feel the doctor communicates with you: reward the doctor who has a good manner and makes you feel comfortable.

Patient notes
- Chris S, age 16
- Usual childhood immunisations
- No significant past medical history

Discussion
The intention for this case is for it to represent a teenager presenting with bone pain from an osteosarcoma. The pain is from the upper tibia rather than the knee joint and is not particularly related to exercise. The main differential diagnosis would be Osgood Schlatter's disease, but this patient's pain is not exercise related, is worse at night and is definitely not located around the tibial tubercle. There are several challenges in this case:

- Communication with a teenager
- Recognising the possibility of a serious illness from the symptoms and signs presented
- Striking a balance between inappropriate reassurance and causing alarm.

How do you communicate with a teenager? Treat them much as you would an adult, with respect. Explore and value their ideas and concerns. Strike the right balance between using language that is easy to understand without being patronising. Teenagers are generally more nervous about communicating with a doctor — as a GP trainee you may feel you are quite young yourself but to a 16 year old you are an old person and very much 'establishment"!

The vast majority of patients we see do not have a serious illness and there is minimal scope for us to cause them harm by inaction. However, most serious illnesses will present to a GP first and you must be alert for warning bells in every consultation. Trainees facing this case on one of my courses commented that they felt it was an unfair case until it turned out that two of the trainees attending the same course had known children in school who had had an osteosarcoma, one of which was mismanaged by her GP with serious consequences! Beware any patient presenting with pain that may be of bony origin that is worse at night.

If you do suspect the serious diagnosis in this case what should you do about it? Obviously you need to investigate or refer this patient but what do you tell him/her? One approach is to be very reassuring, but say that you would like to do an X-ray just to make sure. The other end of the spectrum is to actually tell the patient of your concerns but this is fairly inappropriate for this consultation, especially with no parent present. We often have to arrange investigations for patients where we suspect they may have something serious but feel it is not the right time to articulate your concerns explicitly for fear of causing unnecessary worry. For the case presented here it is probably better to adopt the former approach.

Marking domains

This case is pretty evenly balanced between the domains although as often happens one domain (clinical management) is heavily reliant on another (information gathering) — that is to say that if you do not identify the correct symptoms/signs you will not make the right diagnosis and therefore your clinical management cannot be adequate.

The examiner here will be looking for you at least having a suspicion of a potentially serious diagnosis, so failing to arrange an X-ray or refer the patient would not automatically result in failing the case as long as there was some inkling of your concern and reasonable safety netting, for instance seeing the patient again within a week or two.

6. A request to change treatment

Overview
A patient taking simvastatin asks for his therapy to be changed to atorvastatin while the practice's policy is to use simvastatin.

What the case is designed to test
- Listening to a patient's concerns and negotiate a way forward taking the patient's individual circumstances into consideration
- Managing conflict between a practice's policy and treating a patient as an individual.

Role-player briefing
You are David H, a 65-year-old diabetic who also suffers from hypertension and raised cholesterol. You have been on simvastatin 40mg for your cholesterol for about 10 years and recently heard media reports that a drug called atorvastatin was more effective but that GPs were under pressure not to prescribe this because it was more expensive.

When you saw the practice's nurse in the diabetic clinic recently you spoke to her about it and she said that the practice policy was to use simvastatin unless there were side effects or the cholesterol was not controlled. She said the Local Health Board's prescribing adviser had a 'prescribing incentive scheme' that rewarded doctors for prescribing simvastatin instead of atorvastatin. The nurse said she could not change the prescription and that you would have to see one of the doctors to discuss it. So here you are today.

You have actually been fairly happy on the simvastatin, it seems to be working OK and you have not noticed any side effects, but you are not keen on having an inferior drug on principle. Perhaps your cholesterol would be even better on atorvastatin?

You are on insulin for your diabetes, lisinopril 10mg for your hypertension, aspirin 75mg a day, and the simvastatin. Your diabetes is fine, as is your blood pressure and you really do not want to discuss those today, just the cholesterol lowering drug. If the doctor tries to discuss the other problems get around it politely by saying: '*I'm sure you're very busy doctor and I only really came to talk about the prescription.*'

Opening statement
'*I wonder if I could change my simvastatin doctor?*'

How to behave
You are a well informed, well motivated retired car salesman who takes an active interest in managing his own medical problems. You have a lot of respect for the practice as you have had a good relationship with the doctors and staff for many

years, so although you want to be quite pushy and assertive you do not want to upset the doctor therefore you should do this without becoming angry or irritated. You really do not want to cause this individual doctor any trouble but you cannot see why changing your prescription is going to make a great deal of difference financially. You have looked up the drug costs and know that simvastatin 40mg costs the NHS £17 per year while atorvastatin 10mg costs about £234, therefore the additional cost is just over £200 per year which does not seem much in the overall scheme of things.

If the doctor puts forward some good arguments why your prescription should not be changed then be prepared to accept this, if not then keep pushing!

Patient notes

- David H, age 65.
- 20 years ago: non-insulin dependent diabetes
- 18 years ago: hypertension
- 15 years ago: switched onto insulin
- 10 years ago: started on simvastatin for hyperlipidaemia
- Your practice policy is to use simvastatin as first line, switching only if side effects or inadequate control
- Current therapy: insulin as per specialist nurse guidance (lisinopril 10mg daily; simvastatin 40mg daily; aspirin 75mg daily)
- One month ago diabetic review: Diabetes well controlled, HbA1c 4.9; BP 124/75; Total cholesterol 3.9, LDL 2.1, HDL 1.0, Triglycerides 1.4; HDL: Total cholesterol ratio 26%; asked about atorvastatin instead of simvastatin — practice policy explained.

Discussion

Clearly there are two possible outcomes here, either Mr. Hamilton gets his atorvastatin or not! This case is more about the negotiation than the outcome and the good candidate will establish rapport, ask lots of open questions about his understanding of his therapy, compliment him on his diabetic control and find out exactly what he has read that has led to this request. It is best to avoid being defensive and getting into discussions about the practice's policy or the broader issues around healthcare rationing until later on when you have finished your information-gathering.

There is a real issue here in that drug companies are increasingly targeting the 'consumer' and although they cannot do this directly via advertising they can do so via sympathetically worded articles in the media. Although the additional cost can be looked at as an absolute amount (£200) in percentage terms it is a 13-fold increase in price. Apart from this it would not generally be a good thing for you to undermine the practice policy by acceding to his request.

Does Mr. Hamilton have a point? Well, yes, he might, but given his already excellent control any incremental benefit from switching to a different statin is likely to be minuscule. You can also argue for the *status quo* from the point of view of side-effects and risk. Simvastatin has been on the market for over 20 years and we are very familiar with its adverse effects. Mr. Hamilton himself has been on the drug for 10 years without problems so it seems likely he has more to lose than to gain from a switch to a newer and slightly less well known drug. Of course if he gets his way then why shouldn't any other patient be able to make the same choice? On the other hand this is clearly a highly motivated patient

If you are very persuasive he might come round. If not you might have to negotiate some form of deal with him. In this specific case it might be reasonable for you as a trainee GP to say that you cannot breach the policy without discussion with one of the partners. An alternative might be to accept that since he is a highly motivated patient it would be a pity to adversely affect the doctor-patient relationship over this and perhaps offer him a trial of treatment with an agreement that if there is no measurable improvement within say three months that he will go back to the simvastatin.

For this case, the patient record pretty much gives away what the consultation will be about, giving you the opportunity to do some planning before the patient comes in. You can also look up the drugs in the *British National Formulary* if required.

Marking domains
This case is fairly heavily weighted towards interpersonal skills but with information gathering and clinical management also featuring.

As has already been suggested, the pass/fail decision does not hinge on the prescribing decision. Instead the examiner is looking for a candidate who is sensitive to the patient's request, mindful of the practice policy and conducts a skilful negotiation. Either giving in too easily without putting forward some reasonable arguments or conversely being over-rigid will get you into trouble.

7. Complaint

Overview
A patient consults to make a complaint following a missed diagnosis.

What the case is designed to test
The candidate's ability to adopt a patient centred approach to dealing with the complaint, balancing this with the need not to accept liability on behalf of a colleague.

Role-player briefing
You are John M, and are aged 55. You work as a legal secretary at a local law firm.

Three weeks ago you became unwell. You had a temperature and developed a cough. After a couple of days you rang the surgery and spoke to Dr Wells who said he thought you had a viral infection and that it would most likely clear by itself. You asked about having cough medicine or an antibiotic but he said they were not necessary and advised you to take some paracetamol. Over the next couple of days you became increasingly unwell with severe shivering episodes and a lot of green phlegm. You noticed that you were a little bit out of breath when you climbed the stairs. During the night your wife became worried about you and took you to casualty where the doctor said you had a pneumonia and you were admitted to hospital. You had X-rays and were put on a drip for two days and were allowed home again a couple of days later. You are now feeling much better and plan to start work again next week.

Opening statement
'Hello doctor. I'd like to make a complaint about Dr. Wells.'

How to behave
You have previously been fit and well and in particular have never had any chest problems. You are on no medication. You finished the antibiotics a couple of days after coming home from hospital and the cough settled very soon after that. You now are not coughing, your breathing is normal when you go out walking your dog and although you think you lost a couple of pounds while you were in hospital you have put them back on again. The doctors in the hospital said they were not unduly concerned but that they will see you in the out-patient clinic after six weeks to check your pneumonia has cleared up.

You are upset about Dr. Wells dismissing your concerns when you rang and are pretty sure you would not have had the pneumonia if he had given you some antibiotics.

You are upset and a little angry but try not to let the anger dominate the consultation! You do nor really know what you want out of the consultation, you really came to get it off your chest and you think Dr. Wells ought to know about what happened. You do not plan to take any legal action but don't volunteer this information unless asked.

If the doctor asks you exactly what Dr Wells said, be prepared to admit that he did offer to have a listen to your chest if you were worried but again do not volunteer this without being asked, nor the fact that he said to call back if you got worse. If the doctor asks why you did not call the surgery back when you became more ill say it is because you felt awkward after Dr Wells was a bit dismissive on the phone. At the time you spoke to him about your cough you were not actually feeling terribly ill and you do not think you had a temperature at that stage.

Try to respond to the doctor's approach — if he/she becomes very defensive this will make you a bit more pushy. If he/she appears to be siding with you and agreeing that Dr Wells was wrong acknowledge this and ask what he/she plans to do about it. If he/she offers to arrange an appointment with Dr Wells to discuss your complaint ask who else will be there. If he/she offers to discuss your complaint with Dr. Wells and see you again be prepared to accept this but try to find out exactly what he plans to discuss with Dr. Wells — do not let the doctor use this as an escape clause to get you out of the room early! Be prepared to emphasise your belief that a prescription might have prevented the problem but be prepared to accept a well presented explanation if the doctor tries to explain why prescribing an antibiotic over the phone was not appropriate.

Do not be too unreasonable — if the doctor is empathic and acknowledges your concerns but gives a convincing explanation as to why Dr Wells did what he did then be prepared to accept this.

If the doctor explains the practice's formal complaints procedure either say that you will think about it or that it will not now be necessary depending on how well you feel they have addressed the problem.

Patient notes
* John M, age 55
* No past medical history of note
* No regular medication, no allergies
* 3 weeks ago: telephone consultation with Dr. Wells. Cough 2 days. White/ clear sputum, no blood, etc. Not SOB. Advice regarding paracetamol/fluids. Offered to see in surgery
* 1 week ago: discharge notification. Emergency admission from A/E; R LL pneumonia; treated with amoxicillin; OPD and CXR 6/52

Discussion
Dealing with an angry patient is always challenging, even more so when it is in an assessment. You are likely to have had specific teaching on this and we have already discussed it earlier in this book. They key, as with most of these cases, is to remember to stay relaxed, be patient-centred and address the patient's problem.

Once you have allowed this patient to vent his feelings you need to empathise and acknowledge that they have had an unpleasant experience. You should also check that the patient is now feeling better. It is best to then explain that you would like to ask a few questions so you can be clear about exactly what happened. This needs to be done in a neutral way without either being defensive or implying blame on Dr Wells. As usual start with open questions, but you do need to specifically check that Dr Wells did offer to see the patient in surgery and whether he advised the patient to call back in the event of deterioration.

We speak to and see lots of patients early in the course of an illness, often before there are any abnormal physical signs, so it is inevitable that some will become more ill after we have seen or spoken to them and in these cases we expect patients to contact us again. In this case Mr Morris went to A&E — this usually happens either because they have deteriorated to a point where they feel they need to go to hospital rather than see a GP or because they feel awkward calling the GP. This should be sensitively explored.

The good candidate will establish that at the time of the telephone consultation the patient was not actually feeling terribly ill, and Dr Wells did in fact offer to see Mr Morris and did say to call back if he deteriorated, and that the patient gradually deteriorated over a period of two days without calling back. You should sensitively explain that had he called back it was quite likely that appropriate treatment would have been offered and that it sounds like the pneumonia developed after the telephone consultation. The good candidate will also offer a well-reasoned explanation why prescribing antibiotics or a cough medicine over the phone would not have been a good approach.

Clearly something happened in the telephone consultation that put the patient off calling back. This may have been Dr Wells being a little dismissive and perhaps this is worth clarifying with him.

It may be that after a full discussion and explanation Mr Morris feels happier about the situation. You need to explicitly establish this. If not you need to find out what he would like to do. There are several options as outlined in the role-player briefing: would the patient like to meet with Dr Wells himself; would they prefer you to speak to Dr Wells and get back to them? Would they like you to explain the formal complaints procedures?

Marking domains

This case is predominantly in the interpersonal skills domain although it would be difficult to do well overall without establishing the clear history of what happened and when.

Early adoption of a defensive position justifying Dr Wells' approach without being sufficiently patient-centred will result in a more difficult consultation and potentially lower the candidate's grade. Conversely agreeing that Dr Wells' approach was at fault is inappropriate and could be deemed to be unprofessional if it undermines him. Again, make sure you address the patient's problem

– do not fob the patient off with the practice complaints procedure although an explanation of this certainly should occur.

The examiner will be looking for an empathic but neutral exploration of the sequence of events and following this to guide the patient through the possible alternative ways of trying to find a resolution.

8. Acne

Overview
A teenager presents with acne.

What the case is designed to test
The candidate's ability to consult with a teenager and negotiate a management plan for this common condition involving the patient appropriately.

Role-player briefing
You are Christine W, a 16-year-old and you have just started A levels in college. Since you were 13 you have always had a few spots like everyone else and you have tried Clearasil and a few other things your mum got you from the chemist. Over the last 6 months the spots have been worse — you do get some on your face but most of them are on your upper back with some on your chest. They do tend to fluctuate a bit and since your mum booked the appointment with the doctor a couple of weeks ago they have improved a bit but you fully expect them to get worse again.

Your older brother, David, is 19 and he had spots when he was younger but never saw a doctor. He has a few scars from them on his face and you really do not want to have any scars yourself.

Even though the spots are not too bad you are very self-conscious of them and are very embarrassed about them. Eventually your mum persuaded you to come to see the doctor. You have a boyfriend and are worried the spots will put him off you. A friend at school has bad spots and his doctor gave him antibiotic tablets which seem to have helped

Opening statement
'I've come about my spots doctor'

How to behave
If the doctor asks you to tell him/her more about them say that they come and go a bit and are usually worse on your back and chest, that you have tried a couple of things from the chemist but wait till they ask before telling them about your brother and do not tell them about your friend and his treatment straight away.

If the doctor asks anything about why you think you get them say your mum says eating things like crisps, chips and chocolate make them worse. You have tried avoiding them but do not really think it made any difference. The Clearasil did not seem to make much difference either and in any case you could not reach to put it on your back.

The doctor will probably want to examine you — obviously you (probably!) will not have anything to see on your face so when the doctor asks to examine you the examiner will intervene either with a photograph or a verbal explanation of moderately severe acne.

The doctor may offer you different options — either an antiseptic lotion, an antibiotic lotion or antibiotic tablets/capsules. You are prepared to give the lotion a go but say it is a bit difficult putting it on your back. You really are not keen on your mum or anyone else putting it on for you. Ask how long it will take to work and what else you can try if it does not work. Ask if there are any side effects (say that the Clearasil stings). If you are offered the antibiotics by mouth accept them.

If the doctor suggests referring you to a skin specialist (dermatologist) ask how long that will take (but not if they are suggesting it as an option if the treatment they are offering you does not work).

If the doctor asks to see you with your mum ask why.

If the doctor starts asking any personal stuff about your relationship with your girlfriend, smoking/drinking, safe sex advice, etc. be evasive and say you just want your spots treating. Some doctors may explore the possibility of using the contraceptive pill to control the acne — if they ask about whether you use contraception make it clear you do not use any as you have not had sex with your boyfriend yet.

boyfriend

Patient notes
- Christine W, age 16
- Usual childhood immunisations
- No significant past medical history

Discussion
There are two challenges to this case, firstly the issues around communicating with a teenager and secondly the clinical management of acne. We have already discussed the teenager communication issues in a previous case — treat the patient with respect, try not to patronise.

It may occur to you that this is actually a hidden agenda and that the patient (particularly if the patient is female) may be trying to get oral contraception. It is a reasonable enough suspicion but as you cans see above the role-player is well briefed to head this off quite explicitly, therefore if you ask about contraception and get a negative response take this at face value and do not waste time by continuing to try to explore it.

There is a small part of this case about health beliefs—— how diet affects acne. This is an opportunity for rapport building since it sounds here as if the mother has been nagging the teenager about chips/chocolate, etc. and if you explain that it is nothing to do with their diet it may help them feel you are 'on their side'.

You really must have a coherent management plan for acne; it is a common condition so there is no excuse for not having one in your head. Rummaging around in the *British National Formulary* wastes time and potentially makes you look as if you do not know what you are doing.

You should have a step-wise approach, usually starting with a topical antiseptic, followed by a topical antibiotic and finally an oral antibiotic. In this case patient preference should guide you towards oral therapy — using topical preparations on the back is both practically difficult for the patient and will require relatively large quantities.

Make sure you explain about the treatment you prescribe: how often it should be taken and more importantly how long it might take to work and how long the patient is likely to need to take it. As long as you clearly state to the patient what you are going to prescribe and how they should take it there should not be any need to physically hand over a prescription although it can be a useful way of closing the consultation.

Marking domains

This case is roughly equally split between clinical management and interpersonal skills. It' i probably one of the less challenging cases and you may find you get through it in less than 10 minutes. Do not make it more difficult for yourself by looking for hidden agendas that are not there. Ask if the patient is worried about anything else — if they are they will be briefed to exhibit discomfort, squirm, look down at the floor instead of at you, etc.

The patient-centred doctor will discover that this patient would prefer an oral treatment, and this seems reasonable in view of the distribution of the acne. You may feel strongly that a trial of topical treatment should be first line, and this will be OK so long as it is skilfully negotiated with a clear indication that you will step up to oral treatment if it does not work. The examiner will not mind which particular preparation you decide to use so long as it is an accepted acne treatment. The explanation about the treatment is far more important.

9. Back pain

Overview
A patient presents with straightforward mechanical back pain with no red flag symptoms or signs.

What the case is designed to test
Ability to make a clinical diagnosis, explain the nature and natural history of the problem to the patient and negotiate a realistic management plan.

Role-player briefing
You are Rob R, a 48-year-old in generally good health but for the last few weeks you have had low back pain. You do not particularly remember doing anything to injure your back but it hurts when you bend or move about. It tends to be very stiff first thing in the morning (although it does not keep you awake in the night) and eases off a bit when you are up and about. During the day it stiffens up if you sit or stand for a while. You sometimes get an aching pain in the buttocks when it is really bad but you have had no pain down the legs and no other symptoms.

Opening statement
'I've come about my back doctor.'

How to behave
You have had a bad back lots of times before but it is usually when you have been lifting something heavy. It usually lasts a few days and gets better but over the last few years it has tended to last a bit longer, often going on for a month or six weeks. You have never seen the doctor about it before and you occasionally take a couple of paracetamol for it but you do not like taking tablets very much as you had heard the pain is meant to stop you damaging your back.

You are in good general health and have not lost any weight or noticed anything else. You are married with grown-up children and you work as a delivery van driver for a local motor factor delivering car parts to garages. You do find driving aggravates your back but you really do not want to take time off work unless the doctor thinks it is necessary. You are generally fit and active but the only real exercise you get is cycling once or maybe twice a week. You do not smoke and are a moderate drinker — 4 or 5 pints a night at weekends only.

You should wear casual clothing. You will need to remove your trousers to be examined so wear something that is easy to remove and with shorts underneath.

You are the kind of person who does not go to the doctor often and do not remember the last time you came. You have come this time because the back pain has lasted longer than usual and you are concerned it is getting worse over the years. You wonder if it ought to be looked into a bit further, maybe with an X-ray and you wonder if there is anything the doctor can do to help it get better.

You are not particularly anxious or aggressively pushy but you really would like something doing. You do not have any particular agenda and are open to most suggestions although you will ask the doctor about the benefits of any particular course of action he/she might take. A friend suggested seeing a local private physiotherapist he went to as he manipulated his back and 'put it back in' but you have not done that and thought you would ask the doctor first. If the doctor suggests tablets you want to know if they will actually help the problem clear up and if there is any risk of you damaging your back through doing too much if they take the pain away. If he/she suggests referring to a physiotherapist, osteopath or specialist ask how long the waiting list is. If the doctor does not mention it ask if an X-ray might help. If the doctor does not discuss your work ask at the end if it is OK to carry on working.

The doctor may well want to examine your back. If he/she asks you to bend (e.g. touching your toes) you can only bend about half way before it gets too painful. If you are laying flat you can only lift your legs to about 45 degrees before the pain stops you — the examiner will run through this with you before you play the role. They may want to test the reflexes in your legs so it would be helpful if you are prepared to removed your shoes and socks but you will not be expected to undress any more than this.

There is a balance to be struck between giving too much of the above away too soon and making life too difficult! Just start with the opening statement and see what other questions the doctor asks you. If the doctor asks you open questions (like 'tell me a bit more about the pain') then respond accordingly and reward a doctor who appears interested and makes you feel comfortable.

Patient notes
- Rob R, age 48
- Last consultation 12 years ago for bronchitis. Scattered crackles both lung fields, treated with amoxicillin.

Discussion
This should be a very straightforward case with no hidden tricks or traps. Low back pain is extremely common so you should be very familiar with it. You should be able to identify quickly the lack of any 'red flag' symptoms and be able to offer practical, evidence-based advice to this patient about how to manage it.

Although you could argue that since the patient has no neurological symptoms there is no need to examine for muscle power and reflexes, this would not be a wise approach in the exam. You must at least do a straight leg raising test, assess muscular power (especially dorsiflexion of the big toe) and knee and ankle jerks. This can potentially take up quite a bit of time so you need to be efficient and focused. You can explain your findings as the patient gets dressed again.

You should discover the patient's concerns about having an X-ray, physiotherapy, manipulation, work, etc. and be able to deal with these in a convincing fashion. There is no indication for an X-ray and you should be able to explain this to the patient's satisfaction. The evidence does not really support physiotherapy and in any case it is not likely to be immediately available to you. There is some evidence to support manipulation but in most areas it is not available on the NHS and it is not cheap. There are also issues around qualifications of physiotherapists, osteopaths and chiropractors and I am always concerned when I hear a patient has been told a therapist has 'put something back in'!

You should discuss the role of exercise in helping him overcome his back problem and preventing relapse/recurrence and should offer him sensible advice regarding work. There is quite a lot of ground to cover in 10 minutes so the case is also testing your efficiency, make sure you keep an eye on the time and allow enough time for explanation at the end.

Marking domains
Information gathering is fairly important to this case, but the main emphasis is on the clinical management. A good candidate will be able to address the patient's concerns, give sensible advice about exercise, etc. and will be generally reassuring and encourage the patient to be positive.

Pitfalls include succumbing to the request for an -ray, a clumsy examination and garbled explanation. The examiner is looking for the patient to be leaving the room feeling reassured that he does not have a serious problem and feeling that he has received practical advice on how to manage his problem positively.

Inflammation of plantar fascia.

10. Foot pain

strong band of tissue that stretches from heel to middle of foot bone,

Overview
A patient presents complaining of gradually increasing foot pain.

What the case is designed to test

"Policeman's heel"

- Making an accurate diagnosis through history and examination
- Explaining the diagnosis and offer a sensible range of management options.

Role-player briefing
You are Jim H, a 48-year-old warehouseman. You are married but your children have grown up and left home.

For about three months now you have had a pain in your left foot. You did not injure it — it just came on gradually. The pain is underneath your foot, just in front of the heel and towards the inner side of your foot. It hurts when you put weight on your foot and seems to be at its worst when you first stand on it in the morning. It then hurts when you walk on it but seems to gradually get better over the next couple of hours. The pain has gradually increased, and is now present during much of the day. Once you take your weight off it is OK but hurts again as soon as you stand or walk again.

Your work involves being on your feet for most of the day. You have to wear steel toe capped boots in work. You have not missed any work so far but you are worried that if the pain gets any worse you might have to.

Opening statement
'I've been having this pain in my foot doctor'.

How to behave
Initially just tell the doctor the pain is under your foot without giving away too much detail. The doctor should ask about whether you have injured it, where the pain is, what makes it better/worse, etc.

You have taken paracetamol which helps a bit, but ibuprofen (two 200mg tablets up to three times a day) seems to help more and was controlling it until recently. They are not causing any side effects but you are a bit worried about taking them every day for so long. Lately you are needing to take them to get through the day at work.

If asked you are sure what it might be, but wondered if it might be arthritis. If asked what you thought the doctor might do or what you would like him/her to do you again do not have any particular thoughts but are keen to get it fixed if possible. If asked what your wife thinks say she has not really suggested anything but you think she is getting a bit fed up of you moaning about it.

The doctor may want to see you walk up and down and is likely to want you to remove your shoes and socks to be examined. You should decline any other examination. The examiner will show you where the tender spot on your foot is.

The doctor may (hopefully!) offer you more than one option, for each try to find out the pros and cons:

- Different tablets: are these any better than the ibuprofen? Any side effects? Will they actually cure the problem or just relieve the pain?
- Shoe inserts: are they on prescription or will you have to buy them? Where from, how much?
- A steroid injection: you are not keen on the thought of this and you will give off appropriate non-verbal signs! Will it hurt? Are there side effects? You thought steroids were not a good thing. Will it cure it or just relieve the symptoms? Will one injection work? Who will do it, where and when?
- Physiotherapy: how soon can you get it, how soon will it work?

Other questions to ask:

- Am I going to have this for good?
- Is it a form of arthritis?
- Why have I got it?

Patient notes
- Jim H, age 48
- No significant past medical history

Discussion
Making the diagnosis of plantar fasciitis should be reasonably straightforward but you are looking for a good systematic history and a reasonable examination. There are no specifics to look for in the examination since in reality most experienced GPs will have made the diagnosis on the history and will conduct just a quick examination to confirm the tender spot. Remember the basic principles of all examination: inspect first (look at both feet to compare), check range of movement, etc. then palpate. It is also worth checking the gait is normal.

Explanation of the diagnosis should be in language the patient understands and a good candidate might write the diagnosis down for the patient so he can look it up for himself.

A good candidate will offer the patient several sensible management options and will involve him in a thorough discussion of the pros and cons of each, facilitating shared decision-making. Hopefully the usually self-limiting nature of the problem will be explained.

Be honest about the potential benefits/side effects of whatever drug treatment you might offer. Do not pretend, for example, that giving diclofenac is going to confer a huge benefit over the ibuprofen the patient has been taking, or that a NSAID is likely to actually cure the problem.

If you are going to refer for physiotherapy you should have a rough idea of how the physiotherapist might treat it and also how long the waiting list is (be realistic here and do not suggest the patient will receive treatment within a week if you know you have a three month wait in your own practice).

You need to be able to explain the pros and cons of a steroid injection. This needs to be in plain language that the patient can understand. If you are able to inject plantar fasciitis yourself then it is easy to arrange that, otherwise you might need to explain that you would refer to a colleague.

Do you really feel any one treatment option is clearly better than the others? If so you should say so, otherwise you should be helping the patient to choose between them. If he is uncertain about the injection it might be an idea to suggest he thinks about it and sees you again in a week or so.

Note that much of this discussion could apply to other clinical scenarios. The principles of examination apply to most musculoskeletal examinations and the treatments options are similar to those you might offer for a tennis elbow or a shoulder impingement syndrome.

Marking domains

This case is predominantly in the domains of information gathering and clinical management, although the former should not present too many difficulties and the clinical management is the more challenging part. This being the case it is important not to spend too long on the examination. An experienced GP is likely to make the diagnosis mainly on the history.

The examiner will be looking for a clear explanation of the diagnosis, a reasonable range of treatment options also explained clearly, and a shared decision with the patient.

11. Deafness

Overview
A patient presents complaining of hearing loss.

What the case is designed to test
* Making a clinical assessment of hearing loss
* Giving appropriate advice and/or refer appropriately.

Role-player briefing
You are Tony W, a 48-year-old delivery van driver and your wife has nagged you into coming to the doctor. She says your hearing has been getting worse over the last couple of years — she keeps having to repeat herself to you and is always complaining you have the TV too loud. She is right of course and you are aware that your hearing is not what it used to be. You really struggle to hear conversation when you are in an environment with quite a bit of background noise, like in the local pub. Your wife thinks you should get a hearing aid but the thought horrifies you as you really do not want to be seen out and about with one of those things stuck behind your ear.

You have had no other ear symptoms — no pain, no discharge, no ringing or buzzing. You do not have any dizziness. You think both ears are affected about the same.

Although you work as a delivery driver now you used to work in the Ford Factory where it used to be very noisy. They did provide hearing protectors but not many of you used to wear them as they were hot and a bit uncomfortable.

You are otherwise fit and well and you have never had any serious illnesses.

Opening statement
'My wife thinks I'm going a bit deaf doctor.'

How to behave
You are a bit embarrassed about your hearing, you think it makes you appear a bit stupid and you hate having to keep asking people to repeat what they have said. Although your wife has made you come you do realise there is a problem with your hearing but you probably would not have come of your own accord partly through embarrassment and partly because you do not think there is anything the doctor can do.

You really are not keen on the idea of a hearing aid but you will allow yourself to be persuaded to be assessed in the ear, nose and throat clinic if the doctor makes an effort. If the doctor talks about the miniature 'in ear' aids say you have heard of them but thought they were very expensive.

Be prepared for the doctor to examine your ears — he/she will probably want to look into them with an auriscope and may well want to do a couple of tests with a tuning fork. Just go along with the tests and give truthful answers about what you can hear, etc. Make sure the examiner looks in your ears and tries out the tuning fork tests before playing the role.

You're particularly worried your hearing is going to get worse so ask the doctor if this is the case. If so, ask if there is anything that can be done to prevent it.

Patient notes
- Tony W, age 48
- No significant past medical history

Discussion
This is another clinical management case again with an element of examination in it. Before going to the exam make sure you are familiar with Rinne's and Weber's tests; it is no good simply knowing how to perform them, you must be able to correctly interpret the findings too. The role-player can be trained to respond to simulate either a conductive hearing loss or a sensorineural loss, and bilateral or unilateral abnormalities. Do not assume the patient will have presbycusis, and ignoring signs suggestive of an acoustic neuroma will not go down well with the examiner.

It really is not worth attempting to test the patient's hearing in the consulting room. It takes up time, is hopelessly insensitive, and the fact is that the patient has given you a crystal clear history that his hearing has deteriorated!

Clearly if you suspect any cause other than presbycusis you should refer. If the patient would like to be considered for a hearing aid then he should be referred. There is the added complication here that the patient's occupation may have contributed to his deafness, although he admits that his employers offered hearing protection and he declined to wear it.

Marking domains
This case covers all three domains: you need to take a history and conduct a fluent examination, you need to consider the management options available, and you need to take the patient's views into consideration in deciding what to do next.

When examining the ears remember how you were taught to hold the auriscope and check that you are not causing the patient discomfort. There are several different ways of conducting Rinne's and Weber's tests — stick with whatever you were taught originally and make sure you have revised it before sitting the clinical skills assessment.

There is no need to force this patient into a decision right away about a hearing aid and it is perfectly acceptable to let him go away and think about it.

12. Pre-menstrual syndrome

Overview
A female patient has come for treatment for severe pre-menstrual syndrome.

What the case is designed to test
Ability to take a sensitive medical and social history, exclude psychopathology, and offer sensible evidence-based treatment options.

Role-player briefing
You are Sophie R, a 30-year-old married woman, and over the last couple of years have suffered from increasingly severe pre-menstrual syndrome (PMT). About a week before your period is due you start to become moody and irritable. At the time you do not think there is anything wrong with you and you take it out on your husband, blaming everything on him. Afterwards you realise your husband has done nothing wrong and that it was you. Minor things irritate you and you feel angry all the time. You do feel irritated with your work colleagues work but manage to contain your anger there.

You have no past medical history and your menstrual cycle is quite normal, bleeding for five days every 28 days. Your periods are not particularly heavy and as soon as your period starts your mood lifts and you are back to normal. You and your husband use condoms for contraception. You have tried a couple of herbal treatments and evening primrose oil but nothing seems to help.

You work as the manageress of a cosmetics department in a large department store. Your husband, Martin, is a teacher. You have two children aged 5 and 7 years, and you probably do not plan to have any more but are not absolutely certain of that.

Although your husband has been very understanding he gets very fed up with your moods and you both feel it is important that you get some help. You have been married for three years and have been happily married with no other issues.

If the doctor suggests any kind of examination ask what they would like to examine and why — the examiner will intervene if needs be.

Opening statement
'*I wonder if you can help me doctor? I'm getting terrible PMT.*'

How to behave
It is quite important for this role that you do not give the whole story away at once, also that you do not give the doctor the impression that there might be any underlying depression (for three weeks of the month you are absolutely fine). Your appetite is fine, you are sleeping OK and you have never had any thoughts of self-harm.

You have talked to your friends about it and they have suggested various treatments including going on the pill, an antidepressant and hypnotherapy. This should only be divulged if the doctor asks you sensitively — use your judgement in how much to give away and when, depending on how the doctor makes you feel. If the consultation seems to be nearing its end and some of these options have not been discussed then ask about them directly.

If the doctor offers you several different options ask which he/she thinks best — you do not really have any preference as so long as the treatment works. If the doctor suggests counselling say you are not very keen on that as you want more than just talking treatment, but if the doctor presents convincing arguments why it might be helpful be prepared to accept it.

Patient notes
- Sophie R, age 30.
- Last year: Well woman clinic: non smoker; BP 115/75; smear taken, smear result: normal.

Discussion
This case again spans all three domains: you will need to take a thorough history to exclude depression, you will need to be able to offer some reasonable treatment options, and good interpersonal skills are required to probe into the effects on the patient's life.

In one sense the diagnosis is easy since it is offered by the patient in her opening statement, but candidates sometimes struggle to accept this at face value and seem to be convinced that she has depression. This obviously tends to lead to a poor overall performance in the case. You need to save yourself plenty of time for discussing treatment options so you should not spend long on this, you should be able to exclude depression with a few well chosen questions.

This patient already has a few ideas about possible treatments but they will only be discovered if you ask sensitively. It is best to leave asking her about any treatments she was aware of or had thought of until you have spent some time exploring what is going on and how it affects her, giving you some time to establish rapport — asking too early might be a mistake.

Perhaps the biggest challenge in this case is offering some treatment options. When there are many different options for treating a condition without one standing out as the definitive treatment that often means none of them are terribly effective! This is the case for pre-menstrual syndrome. Over the years many treatments have been put forward, often with persuasive arguments, but generally followed by evidence being published that questions their use. As doctors we will all interpret and present this quite differently — you could take the pessimistic view and explain that although there are lots of treatment options none of them is terribly likely to be effective, or be optimistic and tell the patient that the good news is there are lots of treatments out there to help her! A middle of the road approach is probably best; certainly individual patients will all respond differently and you should explain the options and help the patient choose for herself. While some of the treatments are relatively benign and free of side-effects (e.g. taking vitamin B6) others may have considerable side-effects (e.g. taking the oral contraceptive pill, SSRIs). It is widely assumed by patients that any 'natural' or herbal treatment is automatically free of side effects and we know this not to be true. Exercise on the other hand has other benefits that might increase its worthiness.

Marking domains

There is some important information-gathering here but the emphasis is more on the clinical management options and interpersonal skills.

The good candidate will gather information using open questions, will empathise with the patient, and then spend a short time asking a few closed questions to confirm the diagnosis. Any attempt at examination will be headed off by the examiner stopping you and telling you examination is normal.

The discussion of treatment options should begin with an exploration of any ideas the patient already has. It is important to be honest about side-effects without scaremongering — while some patients given an antidepressant will experience significant side effects many take them with no problems.

The good candidate will make it clear they take the patient's problem seriously and make it clear they will work with the patient over a period of time to try to help. In scenarios like this it helps the patient if you explain that if one treatment does not help they can come back and you can try another.

The main pitfalls in this case are making assumptions about the diagnosis, failure to demonstrate empathy (this is naturally more difficult when you are stressed), having too narrow a range of treatment options, and being either over-pessimistic or over-optimistic about treatment.

13. Convulsion

Overview
A patient presents with a clear history of a first fit.

What the case is designed to test
- Making a clinical diagnosis and arrange appropriate investigations
- Conducting a risk assessment and give appropriate advice.

Role-player briefing
You are Billy C, 45 years old, and yesterday when you were at home with your wife you felt funny and the next thing you knew you were lying on the floor feeling very drowsy and your wife was panicking and checking you were alright. You had been out in the garden and had come in because you felt a bit strange although you cannot put your finger on exactly how it felt. You were sitting in the kitchen having a cup of tea and your wife says she heard a funny noise like a sort of groan and you fell to the floor and were shaking all over. She says you went a bit blue and were frothing at the mouth and were shaking for about a minute or so before it stopped. You then seemed to be unconscious and she could not wake you up for a minute or two. She dialled 999 for an ambulance. When you did wake up you were drowsy and a bit confused. There was also some blood in your mouth and you think you bit the inside of your cheek.

The ambulance soon arrived and the paramedics checked your blood pressure, put an oxygen mask on you and did an ECG. By this time you were quite scared and they said you had had a fit. They took you to A&E where a doctor checked you over but by this time you were pretty much back to normal. The doctor said you had had a fit but that everything seemed OK now and after you had been there for two hours or so they let you home but said to come and see your GP as you would need more tests. They were very busy and did not really tell you much else. They gave you a letter for your GP which you handed in at reception when you arrived.

You have been pretty shaken up by it, you have never had anything much wrong with you before. You have heard of epilepsy but do not know much about it and do not know anyone who has had it.

You are married with grown up kids. You work as a fisherman on a small local trawler and have done this most of your working life. You live in a semi-rural village and need your car to get to work, etc. You drove to the surgery this morning. You do not smoke and do not drink much during the week (the occasional glass of wine) but at weekends you tend to drink quite a bit in your local pub, up to seven or eight pints a night. You had not been drinking the day you had the fit or the night before.

Opening statement
'I had a funny turn yesterday doctor.'

How to behave

You are worried. You are playing the problem down, referring to it as a funny turn when you know it was a fit. You are pretty stoic, have never been ill before apart from appendicitis when you were younger, and very rarely come to the doctor. You want to know if you have epilepsy, if there is any reason this happened, if it is going to happen again, if you need treatment, etc. You are very worried about work — you are all too aware of the risks if you had a fit on the boat — but do not volunteer this unless the doctor asks. You have not considered the implications for driving.

The doctor may want to examine you but the examiner will stop them.

You had a bit of a headache yesterday evening but feel fine today. You are really hoping this can be dismissed as a 'one off' fit and that your life can carry on as normal.

If the doctor says he/she is going to either refer you or arrange some investigation you want to know exactly what investigations, what they are likely to show, how long it will take, etc. React appropriately if the doctor says you cannot drive and/or go back onto the boat — you really do not know how you will cope without your car as you live in a rural village and you have never done anything else but being a fisherman.

You are worried and upset rather than angry. If the doctor uses any words you do not understand be prepared to ask for clarification.

Patient notes

- Billy C, age 45
- 22 years ago: appendicectomy
- Note from A/E yesterday:

    Dear Doctor,

    Your patient attended A&E yesterday after what sounds like a generalised convulsion. He has no previous history of convulsions.

    By the time he arrived in the department he was well with no ongoing complaints. His BP was 128/85 and a full neurological examination was normal. An FBC and U/E were normal but no other investigations were carried out.

    He has been advised to come to see you for further investigations.

    Yours sincerely,

    Dr. J. Jam, SHO

Discussion

This is a challenging case with lots of ground to cover. Before the patient comes in the notes give you the basics of the story so you can spend a minute or two gathering your thoughts and maybe writing a few prompts on the notes. It should be immediately obvious that you must not waste any time at all on non-productive activity.

You must get a clear history of what has happened to the patient — this is a scenario where you need to be more doctor-centred than normal. Obviously allow him to tell his story in his own words, but you then need to efficiently run through your closed questions.

The clinical examination is a tricky area, on the one hand in the absence of any ongoing symptoms there are unlikely to be any physical signs but on the other you will be worried that if you do not examine the patient you will be penalised for this. The examiners have helped you out here by including the note from A&E which documents a normal neurological examination and a normal blood pressure. It would be quite acceptable to check that the patient has no symptoms today, refer to yesterday's examination and say: '*I can see the doctor in A&E examined you thoroughly and found everything was normal so I won't examine you today unless there's anything you're particularly worried about*'. You should also of course advise the patient that he must return if any symptoms do occur. If you attempt to examine the examiner will intervene and tell you there are no abnormal findings.

You really must identify and address the issues of driving and work for this man. It is difficult to imagine a higher risk work environment in which to have a fit! He needs a CT scan and EEG and these are probably best organised via a neurological referral. Sadly, in most areas patients in this situation are not served terribly well and may well have to wait some weeks or even months for investigation or an opinion. If you have a better service in your area then describe your local circumstances.

He is quite a heavy drinker but is it relevant here? Probably not and now probably is not the time to discuss it — you do not have the time and you do not want the negative impact on rapport that telling him he is drinking too much will inevitably have. If you do ask about alcohol it might be reasonable to suggest that it might be something you could have a chat with him about in the future.

This patient will have lots of questions you probably cannot answer. The most important is the question of whether he is likely to have another fit. The evidence suggests patients having a first unprovoked seizure have about a 40% risk of another one in the following two years, so this is not an insignificant risk.

You are unlikely to finish this consultation in time and it is not a consultation that is likely to leave you with the rosy glow of feeling that you have performed well. That is just the nature of the case and it will certainly be the same for everyone.

Marking domains

This case is again very well balanced between all three domains, perhaps with the critical emphasis being on the clinical management, particularly the aspects relating to driving and work. Most of the important clinical information-gathering is done for you but there is some important social information to discover.

While a key principle in the clinical skills assessment is that the examiners will try to avoid deciding your grade on single issues in this case, if you do not identify and address the risks for this patient you will fail. The good candidate will identify the impact this is going to have on this man and empathise accordingly.

could offer rectal diazepam

14. Depression

Overview
A young adult presents with classical symptoms of depression.

What the case is designed to test
Ability to make the appropriate diagnosis, assess the severity, make a risk assessment and negotiate an appropriate management plan.

Role-player briefing
You are Nicola S, a 28-year-old mobile phone salesperson. You work in a call centre for a telecommunications company. The work is fairly stressful — fast paced with pressure to close sales quickly and get onto the next call. You consider yourself good at your job and have actually always enjoyed the work but lately you are finding it a bit of a struggle. You are finding that the stress is getting to you a bit, you are a bit irritable with the customers and your supervisor is not terribly happy with your current call rate. You have always been a confident outgoing person but that has been knocked a bit recently.

You have been feeling generally a bit down for three-four months, some days you feel OK but most days you feel a bit fed up. You tend to have trouble concentrating and seem to have lost a bit of energy. You are sleeping OK but tend to wake up early at about 5am which is not usual for you. You usually like your sport (netball and aerobics) and watching TV but recently you have not really enjoyed it. You have made yourself carry on doing stuff in the hope that you would be able to pull yourself out of the way you are feeling but it does not seem to be working. You used to go out regularly with your friends at weekends but lately found you did not enjoy it and just ended up going home early.

You are single but have a long term boyfriend. Your relationship is fine and there have been no particular problems between you. You have not really discussed how you have been feeling recently as you did not want to worry them.

You have come because you have been feeling like this for quite a while — you initially thought it would pass and that you could pull yourself out of it but nothing you have tried seems to have helped and you now wonder if you might be depressed and need some help to get better.

Opening statement
'I think I might be a bit depressed doctor.'

How to behave
If the doctor asks open questions start by telling them about work. Do not give too much away initially, wait until the doctor asks you specific questions before telling them about your boyfriend, the early morning waking, not enjoying sport/ socialising, etc.

The doctor is likely to probe for possible causes. Although you are struggling a bit with work you do not think work is really the problem, it is just that you are not performing very well at the moment because of how you are feeling. Likewise with your relationship is fine and you are confident that is not the cause. Do not volunteer all this, wait till the doctor asks you. There are no other social or family problems in your life and you really cannot think why you are feeling like this. You do drink but not very much, you still go out with your friends at the weekend but only have two or three drinks.

The doctor is likely to ask about how depressed you have felt and whether you have thought about harming yourself. Although you feel depressed enough to come to see the doctor you have not been tearful and you have had no thoughts of harming yourself. You are not feeling particularly anxious and are eating OK, you have not gained or lost any weight.

If the doctor asks you about what treatment you had thought about say that you did not really have any particular thoughts about it and are open to suggestions. You do definitely want some treatment though. When the doctor discusses treatments ask about how effective they are, how long they take to work, if they have any side effects. You do not want any treatment that might be addictive or that might interfere with your work. If the doctor suggests counselling ask how long it will take to get an appointment and how quickly it works. If the doctor presents you with various options try to get the doctor to make a recommendation — you do not know much about these treatments and even though you want to know about them you are fairly happy for the doctor to decide on the best plan.

Try to play the role with a fairly flat affect — you are not desperately depressed and have not felt tearful, etc. Speak a little slowly, do not be too garrulous and do not make too much eye contact. You are actually a bit embarrassed about how you feel and about coming to see a doctor about it.

Patient notes
- Nicola S, age 28
- Last smear: Well Woman Clinic. Smear taken: normal. BP 118/72

Discussion
This really should be a straightforward consultation similar to lots of consultations you have done in your own surgery previously. The problem is that when the examiners present you with something terribly challenging they make allowances when you run out of time or do not pick everything up. When it is a common and important general practice problem however they are going to expect you to do it well and you need to get this one right.

You must be patient-centred and acknowledge the patient's embarrassment about coming to you and reassure them that they were right to come. Similarly patients often spend a lot of time worrying about what they have done to bring this on themselves, why they have not been able to pull themselves out of it, etc. and the good candidate will give an appropriate explanation and reassurance.

You need to give practical suggestions as to what they can do to help themselves but emphasise that they also need some help in the form of treatment.

Counselling and in particular cognitive behavioural therapy (CBT) might help this patient but for this scenario where there are no obvious precipitating factors and the patient has already made sensible efforts to overcome the problem. Many doctors feel an antidepressant might offer faster and more reliable benefit especially when counselling could have a lengthy waiting list and CBT often is not available at all.

If you prescribe, the actual antidepressant you choose is not terribly critical, stick to what you know to avoid rummaging through the *British National Formulary*. Do warn the patient not to expect improvement for two to three weeks although it is sensible to arrange to review the patient sooner to make sure they are getting on OK with the medication. It is best to pre-warn them of the common side effects of whatever you prescribe.

Marking domains

You need to cover all three domains in this case. The diagnosis is fairly obvious and is not so dependent on critical information from the history, but safe and effective clinical management is important as are good interpersonal skills.

You really must make an explicit risk assessment in this case.

A good explanation of treatment is key if prescribing antidepressants where the benefits are not immediately obvious and many patients experience side-effects which then often improve over a relatively short time period.

Time management is also important as it is easy to spend too long discussing the symptoms and their effect on the patient's life — while this is important if it prevents you getting to the part of the consultation where you actually prescribe it could be costly. The examiner can only mark what they see and cannot assume that because you appeared to be competent taking a history, made the correct diagnosis and were empathising nicely you would then manage the problem appropriately.